better back

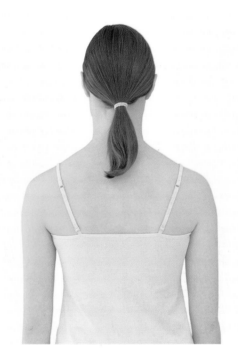

D1211538

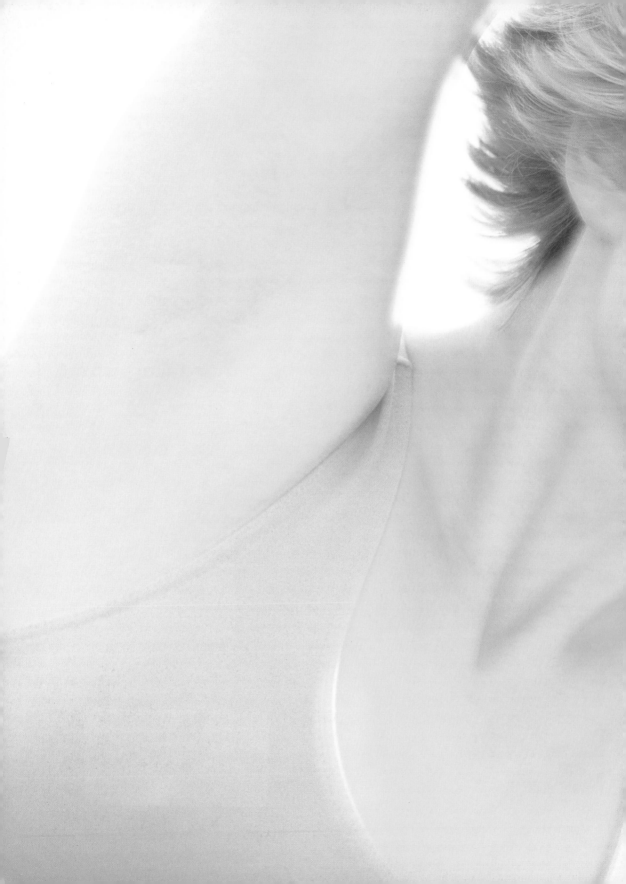

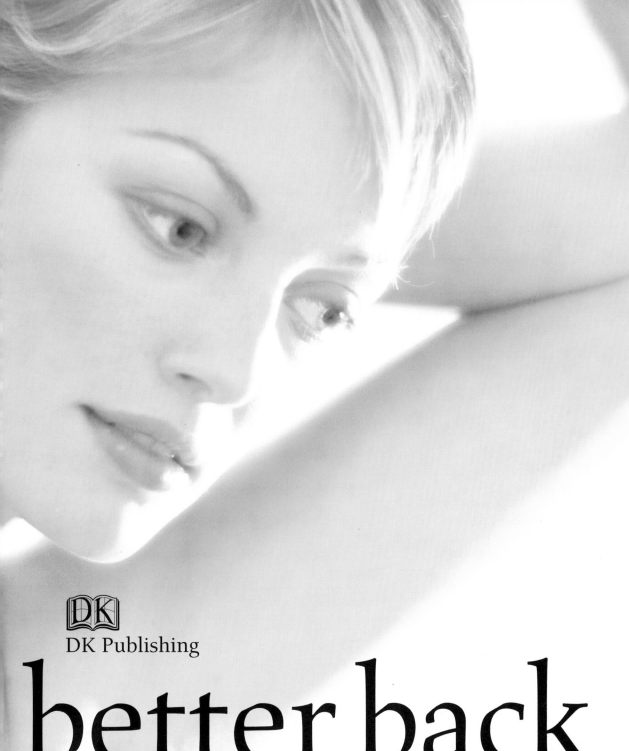

DK Publishing

better back

DR. JOHN TANNER

LONDON, NEW YORK, MUNICH,
MELBOURNE, DELHI

*To Petra, my lovely wife, who reminds me that it
is not only backs that need attention and love.*

US Project Editor: Barbara Berger
Americanizer: Jane Perlmutter
US Medical Consultant: Dr. David A. Lenrow

Project Editor: Pip Morgan **Project Designer:** Jo Grey
Senior Editor: Penny Warren
Managing Editor: Stephanie Farrow
Managing Art Editors: Mabel Chan, Sarah Rock
DTP Designer: Sonia Charbonnier
Production Controller: Louise Daly
Photographer: Ruth Jenkinson

Important notice
Do not try self-diagnosis or attempt self-treatment for
serious or long-term problems without consulting a
medical professional or qualified practitioner. Do not
undertake any self-treatment while you are undergoing a
prescribed course of medical treatment without first
seeking professional advice. Always seek medical advice if
symptoms persist. Do not exceed any dosages
recommended without professional guidance.

Published in the United States by
DK Publishing, Inc.
375 Hudson Street
New York, NY 10014

First published in Great Britain in 2003 by
Dorling Kindersley Limited

Penguin Group
2 4 6 8 10 9 7 5 3 1

Library of Congress Cataloging-in-Publication Data
Tanner, John (John A.), 1952–
Better Back : a self-help guide to preventing and treating back pain with
orthodox and complementary medicine / John Tanner
p. cm.
ISBN 0-7894-9656-9 (alk. paper)
1. Back--Care and hygiene. 2. Backache--Treatment. I. Title.

RD771.B217T36 2003
617.5'64--dc21
2003046258
ISBN 0-7894-9656-9

Reproduced in GRB Editrice, Italy
Printed and bound by Printer Portuguesa, Portugal

Discover more at **www.dk.com**

Contents

Foreword

Back pain affects four out of five people and can be an upsetting experience. The good news is that most people with back pain will get better – but there are important steps to take for a more rapid recovery. John Tanner has written a practical, user-friendly book for people with back pain, which is also an uncomplicated reference for physicians and rehabilitation therapists who want to advise patients.

Better Back helps people understand commonly used medical terms and guides them through the various treatments available. Most importantly, it provides advice to help people to manage their condition themselves. John Tanner encourages people not to take back pain lying down – since research clearly shows those who are active or return to their regular activities as soon as possible tend to recover faster than those who have prolonged rest, or who have become fearful about their condition. John's approach to back pain is a holistic one. There is still much more research needed to determine what treatment options are more effective than others. The healthcare system has tended to keep different types of healthcare professionals apart. We need research into a more collaborative model of healthcare – one that builds on the strengths of each of the various disciplines.

This is one book that I will keep in my library for patients, as well as in the library of the healthcare facilities of those industries for which I consult.

Jack Richman MD

Past Director, American College of Occupational and Environmental Medicine; Founder, Ontario Society of Occupational and Environmental Medicine, Past President, Canadian Society of Medical Evaluators

Introduction

Back pain is one of the most common afflictions in the industrialized world: about 80 percent of the population in developed countries suffer from backache at some time in their lives. This book is addressed to all those who are currently suffering from back pain, and to anyone who wants to take preventive measures to minimize their chances of suffering from a back problem in the future. It may also be of use to therapists who want to know what kind of advice they should give to their patients, or who would like more information on available treatments for back pain.

The book digs deeper than other books. Not only does it explain the causes of back pain in clear, nontechnical terms, it also offers practical advice on how to cope when you have a back problem, describes what to expect when you seek professional help, and gives a thorough assessment of the various therapies available.

Finding the right approach

Back pain is a field with many changing theories and differing professional viewpoints. I have tried to sort out what is hard fact about back pain and its treatment, what is probable, and what is speculation about the benefits of various therapies.

This book takes a holistic approach to back pain and also acknowledges that there are many ways of managing back trouble. Seek out the approach that works for you and don't be put off by such off-hand statements as "nothing can be done," "you have arthritis – learn to live with it" or "you have nonspecific back pain."

Unfortunately, however, it is extremely difficult to predict how quickly anyone will recover from a backache. If the phrase "such and such treatment

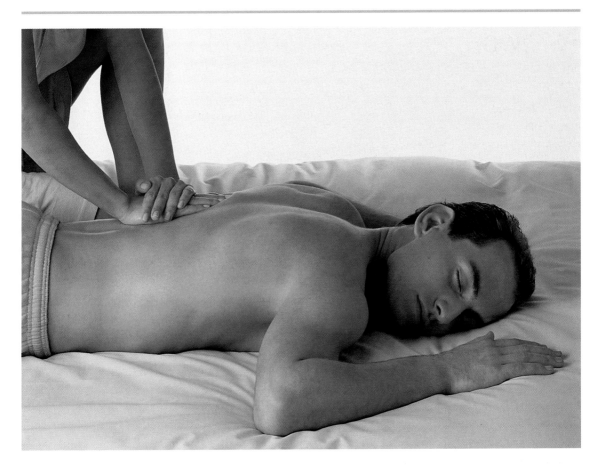

may help in this condition" creeps into this book now and again, it is either because there is no hard evidence regarding the success of the treatment, or because the disorder responds so variably to different treatments as to be quite unpredictable.

Holistic medicine treats individuals, not conditions, and therefore every case is unique. This principle is a theme which runs through this book. The holistic practitioner, whether doctor, nurse, physical therapist, or complementary therapist, never loses sight of his patient as a person: he never isolates symptoms from his patient's general health and mental state.

The therapist's attitude toward you is only part of the story, however. Your attitude toward him is probably equally important. If you trust your therapist, your chances of responding are much higher than if you have little faith in his ability. Even more important are your own attitudes and beliefs about pain, illness, and disability.

Back trouble is not just a mechanical fault to be fixed. Its solution involves correct use, good posture, freedom from tension, and a healthy attitude. No single approach necessarily provides all the answers. In the end, the most helpful approach is one that teaches you how to care for your back so you can become independent of therapy.

John Tanner

1

The
Healthy Back

The spine is a superb and fascinating piece of engineering. It is the central support system for the entire body and plays a role in almost all our movements. In addition, it supports and protects the spinal cord. A healthy back is one in which the spine is firm enough to support the body weight when standing erect, yet strong and flexible enough to provide a steady anchorage and a source of movement of the upper and lower limbs. On top of all this, your spine must provide a safe and cushioned channel for nerves.

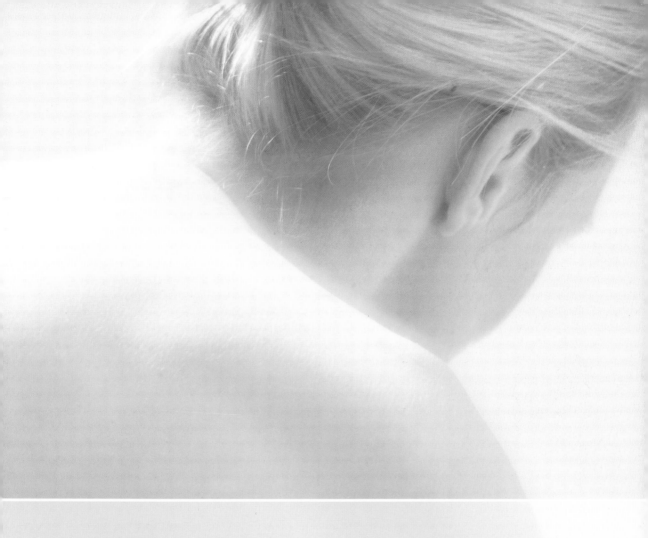

To achieve a healthy back, every part of the spine – bones, joints, disks, ligaments, muscles, and nerves – must work in unison, each contributing stability, power, movement, strength, or flexibility. Most of the time we walk, stretch, carry, make love, or drive a car without worrying about our backs. Yet if you do suffer from back pain, remember that most back sufferers – given a little patience, support, and the right treatment – can return to the happy state of relying on a healthy back.

The spinal column

The spine's column of bones is the central support for the skeleton. The skull is supported chiefly by the cervical and upper thoracic vertebrae. Each thoracic vertebra is joined to a rib on either side – the resulting ribcage surrounds and protects the heart, lungs, and liver. The basin formed by the sacrum and the two iliac bones – the pelvis – protects the organs of the lower body. The spine is a very mobile structure: it can bend and rotate in almost any direction. The cervical and lumbar regions are the most mobile – movement in all directions in the thoracic region is restricted by the rib cage.

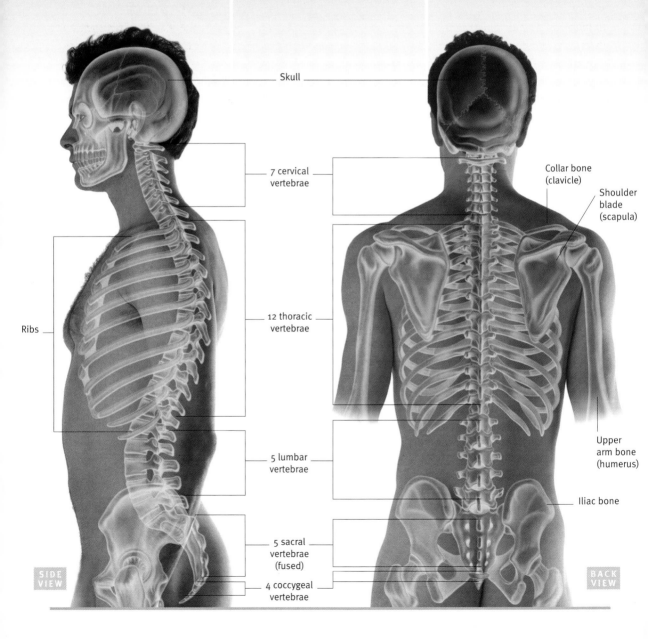

Skull

7 cervical vertebrae

Collar bone (clavicle)

Shoulder blade (scapula)

Ribs

12 thoracic vertebrae

5 lumbar vertebrae

Upper arm bone (humerus)

Iliac bone

5 sacral vertebrae (fused)

4 coccygeal vertebrae

SIDE VIEW

BACK VIEW

The spine

The human spine is a column of up to 34 bones, or vertebrae. All but ten are movable and are divided into three groups: 7 cervical (neck), 12 thoracic (chest) and 5 lumbar (lower back). The base consists of five fused segments called the sacrum, which adjoins one iliac bone on each side to make up the pelvis. Below this we have between three and five (most of us have four) fused or partially mobile segments which form the coccyx, the rudimentary tail that is our primate inheritance.

The structure of a vertebra

The main part of a vertebra is more or less cylindrical, with flat surfaces at the top and bottom. To the back of this main section of the vertebra is a hole, and when the vertebrae are stacked up, these holes form a continuous channel – the spinal or neural canal – which contains the spinal cord.

Behind the spinal canal each vertebra has seven projections, known as processes. They form three pairs with an odd one out, the spinous process. You can feel the spinous processes as knobbly bits all the way down your back.

The three pairs of processes lie to the right and left of this spinous process. Two of the pairs – the upper articular processes and the lower articular processes – act as joints to link the vertebrae together and strengthen the spine. The back muscles are attached to the remaining pair, the transverse processes, and also to the spinous process, all of which provide anchorage as the muscles contract and relax.

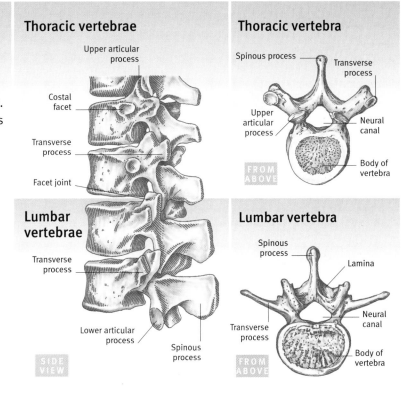

Vertebrae

No two vertebrae are exactly alike. Although they fit together perfectly, they all have individual characteristics. Shown here are cross-sections of the lowest two thoracic vertebrae, which have small flat costal facets where they are attached to the ribcage and the first two lumbar vertebrae, which have much larger spinous processes.

Thoracic vertebrae

Upper articular process
Costal facet
Transverse process
Facet joint

Lumbar vertebrae

Transverse process
Lower articular process
Spinous process

SIDE VIEW

Thoracic vertebra

Spinous process
Transverse process
Upper articular process
Neural canal
Body of vertebra

FROM ABOVE

Lumbar vertebra

Spinous process
Lamina
Neural canal
Transverse process
Body of vertebra

FROM ABOVE

Facet joints

The upper articular processes of one vertebra link up to the lower articular processes of the vertebra above. These processes have flat, smooth surfaces, rather like the facets of a diamond, hence their name, facet joints. They are also known as zygo-apophyseal joints.

Where the smooth surfaces meet they are said to articulate. The articulating surfaces of the facet joints are lined with cartilage and lubricated with synovial fluid. The whole joint is contained within a capsule. Regular and repetitive movement is essential for healthy cartilage and helps to keep the joints working efficiently.

Disks

The flat surfaces on the top and bottom of the main body of the vertebra is covered in a thin layer of cartilage called an end plate. Each vertebra is further separated from the vertebra above and

Spinal joints

The joints between the vertebrae are made of two main elements: a disk that works like a ball bearing to allow the spine to twist and bend (*see p. 13*) and acts as a shock absorber; and facet joints that form a fulcrum (*below*).

Disk structure

Disks contain an outer annulus fibrosus, which is composed of layers of concentric fibers and an inner nucleus pulposus, made of a pulpy gelatinous substance.

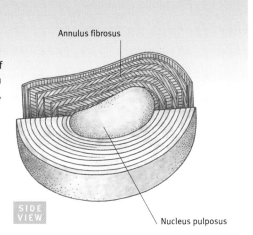

Annulus fibrosus

Nucleus pulposus

SIDE VIEW

The whole motion segment

When the spine bends backward or forward, the facet joint allows a pincer movement to be made. The joint is cushioned by the disk.

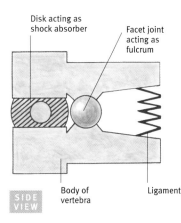

Disk acting as shock absorber

Facet joint acting as fulcrum

Body of vertebra

Ligament

SIDE VIEW

Facet joint structure

The articular processes of a facet joint are lined with protective cartilage. The membrane surrounding the joint secretes a lubricating fluid.

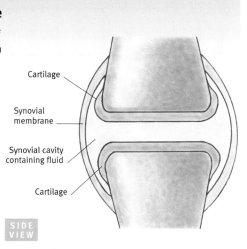

Cartilage

Synovial membrane

Synovial cavity containing fluid

Cartilage

SIDE VIEW

below by a cartilage pad, or disk. The outer layers of the disk, called the annulus fibrosus, are formed from tough fibrous cartilage. The annulus fibrosus blends with the end-plate cartilage around the edge of the vertebrae. Inside the annulus is a gelatinous substance known as the nucleus pulposus. This gel allows the disk to mold itself like a liquid ball bearing, so that in addition to acting as a joint, the disk performs a second equally vital function as a cushion between each vertebra.

The healthy disk is extremely strong – stronger than the bone of a vertebra. It has to be in order to absorb shocks. When compressed, the disk has a breaking strength of 1760lb (800kg) in young people and 990lb (450kg) in the elderly. The disk can absorb compressive and jarring forces very efficiently, distributing loading forces by adapting its shape. It is, however, more susceptible to stresses caused by twisting motions, and the outer layers can rupture.

The annulus fibrosus has few pain-sensitive nerves. The pain associated with a "slipped disk" (a misnomer, since a disk cannot slip) often comes from an injured disk pressing on the dural sheath of the spinal cord or a nerve, or directly from a tear in the annulus fibrosus.

The disk is largely water – 90 percent in babies and 70 percent in a 70-year-old. Repetitive but not excessive exercise encourages a good balance of fluid to fiber, and helps to keep drying out and degeneration at bay.

Disks need adequate periods of rest from the weight of the upper body pressing down. A disk can shrink by ten percent of its height during the day, so you are slightly taller in the morning than in the evening – as much as 0.8in (2cm) overall. A night's rest enables the disk to reabsorb nutrition and fluid through the end plates of the adjacent vertebrae, and regain the height lost over the day.

How the disk allows movement

If you think of the vertebrae in a spinal joint as two pieces of wood and the nucleus pulposus as a soft rubber ball bearing, as shown, it is easy to see why the disk forms such a mobile joint.

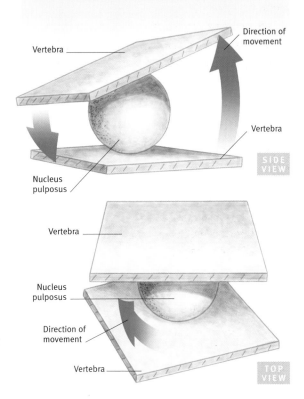

Vertebra

Direction of movement

Vertebra

SIDE VIEW

Nucleus pulposus

Vertebra

Nucleus pulposus

Direction of movement

Vertebra

TOP VIEW

The spinal canal

The vertebrae form a continuous channel called the spinal canal, through which the spinal cord runs. The cord is a bundle of nerves linking the brain with nerves in the body, relaying information to and from the brain. It runs from the base of the skull down to the lumbar vertebrae.

Three membranes, or meninges, surround the spinal cord. The outermost is a sheath called the dura, which extends as far as the second of the

The spinal cord

The spinal cord is continuous with
the brain stem, and finishes at the
first or second lumbar vertebra.
Below this, the nerves run out in
strands which, due to their
appearance, are called cauda
equina, meaning horse's tail. The
cord is surrounded and protected
by the same three membranes
that protect the brain.

Spinal nerves

These emerge in pairs from either
side of the spinal cord through the
foramina, or gaps between the
vertebrae and the facet joints.

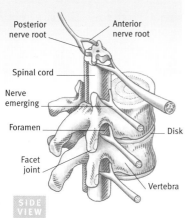

Posterior nerve root

Anterior nerve root

Spinal cord

Nerve emerging

Foramen

Disk

Facet joint

Vertebra

SIDE VIEW

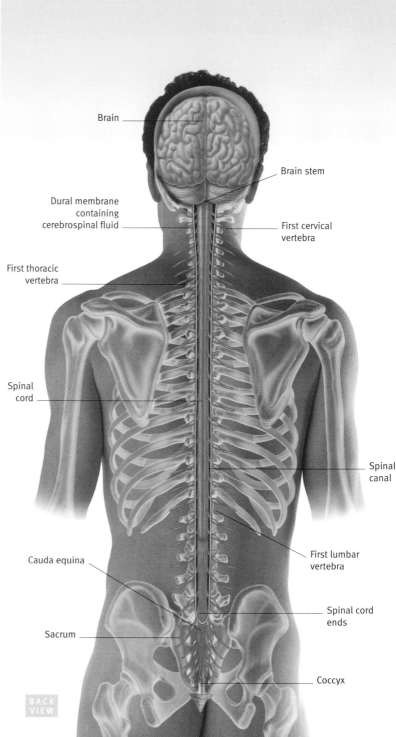

Brain

Brain stem

Dural membrane
containing
cerebrospinal fluid

First cervical
vertebra

First thoracic
vertebra

Spinal
cord

Spinal
canal

Cauda equina

First lumbar
vertebra

Spinal cord
ends

Sacrum

Coccyx

BACK VIEW

sacrum's five fused bones. At the points where the pairs of nerve roots emerge from the spinal cord through the foramina (gaps in the vertebral column), pairs of dural root sleeves project from the dural sheath to enclose and protect them.

The dural sheath is extremely responsive to pressure throughout its length. The dural sheath and root sleeves are quite mobile, but bending or stretching movements can cause the nerve root sleeve to rub against a vertebra, which explains why stretching the nerve in the leg-lifting test can cause pain if you have a disk protrusion (*see p. 36*).

Inside the dural sheath, between the two inner meninges, is the cerebrospinal fluid. This bathes the spinal cord and is continuous with the fluid surrounding the brain. It acts as an extra shock absorber to protect the sensitive spinal cord.

The ligaments

Joints are supported by tough, slightly elastic bands of fiber. These ligaments help hold the bones together firmly and strengthen the small joints at each segment where one vertebra meets another. In combination with the facet joints, the ligaments keep the spine in one piece, allowing only a limited range of movement in any one direction, according to their length. Most of them are richly supplied with nerve endings.

The main ligaments run down the length of the spine at the back and front, while others bind and strengthen the joints. The joints require regular movement otherwise the ligaments will eventually become stiff or weak. Once this has happened, whether through aging, disuse, or tissue scarring, it is difficult to restore them to their original condition. At the same time, they can also become overstretched and slack.

The muscles

Around each joint there is a group of muscles. Each end of a muscle is firmly attached to a different bone, either directly or by means of a band of tissue known as a tendon. Muscles tend to work in pairs: when one muscle contracts, its opposite number relaxes, allowing movement. Close to the joints of the vertebrae many small muscles provide subtle alterations of movement when they contract. These are called stabilizer muscles because they control spinal posture.

Spinal ligaments

A complicated network of ligaments holds all the spinal joints together. The ligaments around the main body of the vertebrae, the anterior and posterior ligaments, extend right down the column to support it.

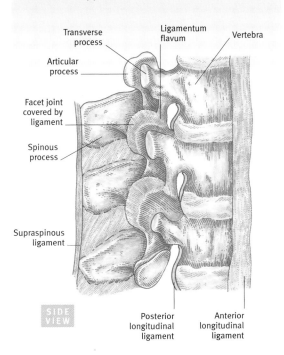

Transverse process

Ligamentum flavum

Vertebra

Articular process

Facet joint covered by ligament

Spinous process

Supraspinous ligament

SIDE VIEW

Posterior longitudinal ligament

Anterior longitudinal ligament

The large muscles

More superficially visible in a lean person are the longer, larger, and stronger muscles that control the major movements of the trunk. They are known as the mobilizers. Muscles known as the erector spinae (literally, "spine raisers") are at the back. They lengthen when you bend over, resisting the force of gravity, and contract even more strongly on straightening, thereby exerting great compressive force on the spine.

Across the front of the body, and also at the sides, abdominal muscles help to support the spine by maintaining pressure inside the abdomen and chest. This pressure provides an essential measure of countersupport to the spine. For example, a professional weight lifter will hold his breath and tense his abdominal muscles in order to lift a heavy weight. The transversus abdominis (the deepest layer) should work almost continually in everyday activities.

How nerves stimulate muscles

The nervous system is made up of millions of nerve fibers, which transmit electrical impulses to and from the brain and connect the brain with the rest of the body. The nerves are divided into two types: sensory fibers, which send signals, such as pain messages, to the brain; and motor fibers, which relay messages from the brain to the muscles. Bundles of muscle fibers are controlled by impulses from the nerves.

When you decide to bend your arm, for example, the brain sends out a message which is transmitted along the appropriate nerves to your biceps, the muscle in the upper arm. This signal makes the biceps contract, which pulls your forearm up, bending your arm at the elbow.

How the muscles move the trunk

When you twist or rotate your spine, the back and abdominal muscles play an important role. Think of the golf player who needs to create a strong twisting force to effect a good drive. This has to be balanced by an equal and opposite twisting movement which is transmitted through the spine and the lower limbs.

Superimposed over the muscles of the back are the muscles that control and move the shoulder girdle and the hip girdle. The muscles supporting your hip joints are very large and strong and form the contours of the buttock and hip. The deeper layers of muscles are smaller and exert a rotating force on your hip joints.

Maintaining healthy muscles

The fibers in muscles have to be able to contract and shorten – some can contract to a third of their original length. When relaxed, they can also be stretched and are therefore elastic to some extent.

Your muscles need a good supply of blood and energy. If the blood supply is reduced – perhaps because a muscle has gone into protective spasm in reaction to pain, or has become chronically contracted due to poor posture – the muscle cells will suffer and their function will be impaired. If this state of affairs continues for long enough, the muscle or muscles become painful, weak and less elastic, and will eventually shorten.

Like ligaments, muscles need regular work and exercise to maintain their strength and encourage healthy local circulation. Muscles that have been contracted for long periods to maintain a certain posture – for example, if you have been sitting down, writing, or typing – need regular stretching to prevent them becoming shorter and weaker.

Excessive nervous system stimulation – such as that which might be caused by pain from an

The muscles of the back

This diagram will give you an idea of how the layers of muscle in the back are built up. The right side of the body shows the various small muscles, those mainly concerned with postural adjustment; the left side of the body shows how the larger muscles involved in movement are laid over the top.

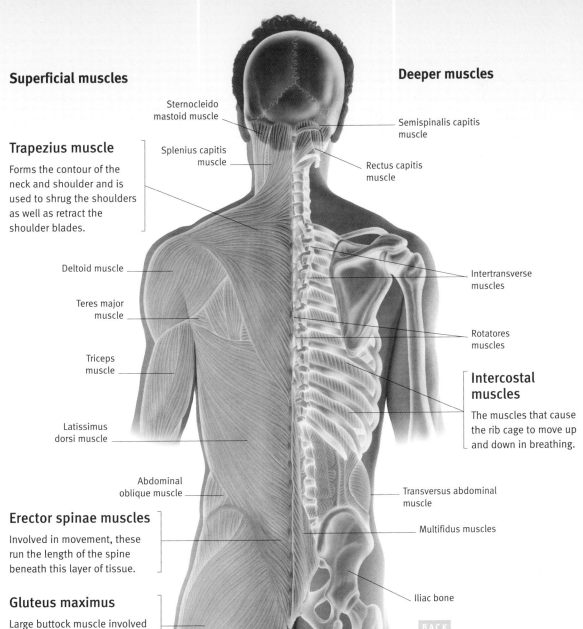

Superficial muscles

Deeper muscles

Trapezius muscle

Forms the contour of the neck and shoulder and is used to shrug the shoulders as well as retract the shoulder blades.

Sternocleido mastoid muscle

Splenius capitis muscle

Semispinalis capitis muscle

Rectus capitis muscle

Deltoid muscle

Teres major muscle

Triceps muscle

Latissimus dorsi muscle

Intertransverse muscles

Rotatores muscles

Intercostal muscles

The muscles that cause the rib cage to move up and down in breathing.

Abdominal oblique muscle

Transversus abdominal muscle

Erector spinae muscles

Involved in movement, these run the length of the spine beneath this layer of tissue.

Multifidus muscles

Gluteus maximus

Large buttock muscle involved in standing and walking.

Iliac bone

BACK VIEW

Psoas muscles

A large group of muscles in the abdomen, the psoas are attached at one end to the transverse processes of the lumbar vertebrae, and are anchored at the other end on the upper part of the thigh bone. The psoas muscles are involved in flexing the hips – for walking or climbing stairs, for example – and play an important role in maintaining posture for sitting.

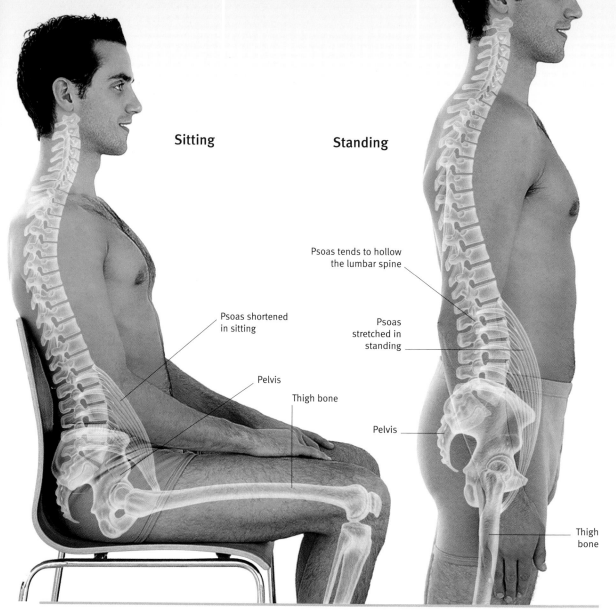

Sitting

Standing

Psoas tends to hollow the lumbar spine

Psoas shortened in sitting

Psoas stretched in standing

Pelvis

Thigh bone

Pelvis

Thigh bone

injury or even by accumulated tension – can make the muscles in the back tense up. Relaxation is therefore another important ingredient in the recipe for maintaining healthy muscles.

Finally, an intact nerve supply is essential to healthy muscles. If, as a result of an injury or an infection such as poliomyelitis, a nerve is severed or its cell body in the spinal cord is damaged, the muscle cannot contract and will waste away.

Functions of the spine

For all intents and purposes, the structure and function of the spine are virtually identical in all mammals. One significant difference is that, during evolution, our center of gravity has shifted so that the force of gravity exerted on an upright human pulls vertically throughout the length of the body. As a consequence, the human spine, together with its muscles and ligaments, has become a vertical shock absorber, with curvatures to provide the necessary resilience.

The spine is not just a rigid support system, however. Its structure is essential to walking and many other movements. We walk not only with our legs, but with our whole back, and we reach for, grasp, and carry objects not just with our arms but also with our back.

In order to understand how all the separate and intricate parts of the back interrelate, it is useful to think of each area of the spine – the neck, midback, and lower back – in relation to its function.

Movement in the neck

Your neck must be strong enough to hold your head, which is a considerable weight – an adult's head can weigh as much as 14 to 20lb (6 to 9kg). It must also be sufficiently flexible to allow you to turn your head so you can look and listen.

At the same time, you must be able to maintain a level gaze so as not upset your organs of balance. Located deep in each inner ear, these delicate organs are finely tuned to the forces of gravitation and rotation. We achieve this steady gaze through complex feedback mechanisms in the neck muscles and these organs of balance, which allow the brain to account for movement while, at the same time, interpreting visual information.

Movement in the midback

The thorax, or chest, which includes the ribs, allows the movement entailed in breathing. When you inhale fully, the thoracic spine extends slightly as the ribs rise, and when you exhale, the thoracic spine flexes. When you turn the trunk of your body, it rotates around the thoracic spine.

Movement in the lower back

The lumbar region lies below the thoracic part of the spine and must be solid and very strong to support the weight of the upper half of your body. It must also be flexible so that you can bend and reach the ground. (Bending forward from the thoracic spine is necessarily more limited because it would restrict your capacity to breathe by preventing expansion of the lungs.)

The pelvis, including the fused sacrum, must provide a firm base for your abdomen. The pelvis transmits the forces from your spine to your legs through your hip and sacroiliac joints. This downward force counteracts the shock wave which comes up from each foot and leg when you walk or run and which is transmitted through the hip joint and sacroiliac joint into the spine. Some of this force is counterbalanced across the pubic arch of the pelvis, but this whole area must withstand these frequent shearing or asymmetrical forces, reducing the load on the spine.

2

Back Trouble

If you have suffered from back trouble in the past, or you are in pain right now, you have probably asked "Why me?" You may be able to recall some awkward twisting motion or straining action that set off the pain. But why has it happened at this particular time? The chances are that your back was already in a condition where a relatively minor incident was sufficient to trigger a back problem and the associated pain, somewhat like a rope that has been gradually fraying and is then snapped by the slightest tug.

It is difficult to isolate any particular feature which predisposes people to back trouble, but factors such as age, occupation, and fitness all play a part. A study of twins in Finland showed that genetic factors also play a role. This means that you may be predisposed to suffer from back problems regardless of your job or leisure activities due to weaker disk fibers and early degeneration. Since this inherited factor is beyond your control, it is even more important to consider the risk factors that you can control.

Who is most at risk?

Surveys and statistical reports from around the world reveal certain common findings about who is most at risk from back trouble.

Vulnerable age groups

You are most likely to have back trouble between the ages of 30 and 50. Fewer people under 18 and over 60 are affected. The reason for this is likely to be a combination of factors.

The social and occupational demands of the middle years are perhaps the most intense – from raising small children and labor-intensive work to reduced sports or leisure activities and a tendency to gain weight. Disks are most vulnerable between the ages of 30 and 50. Young people have strong, resilient disks, while elderly people have dried out disks composed mostly of inelastic fiber.

Male or female – the weaker sex?

Women seem to be slightly more prone to back trouble than men. The cause for this is not known, but pregnancy, childbirth, and child rearing may take their toll on the spine. Men take more time off work because of back trouble but this may reflect the type of work they do. In addition, men are twice as likely to undergo back surgery.

Posture

Poor posture accounts for a high proportion of back pain. When we talk about poor posture, we often really mean inelegant posture – slouching in a chair or walking with hands in pockets. But no evidence suggests such habits increase the risk of back problems. However, other types of poor posture are a major cause of backache and back trouble. These include: leaning over a desk or working with your arms raised for a long time; lifting heavy weights while bending from your waist instead of at your knees; sitting in a chair of the wrong height or without adequate back support. (*See also Chapter 8.*)

Fitness and strength

Research suggests that insufficient exercise increases the risk of back problems. If you are fit, your muscles will be strong and flexible, and you will recover more quickly from any injury or illness than an unfit person. Your bones will be stronger, too. If you remain fit as you grow older, your bones will retain their strength longer.

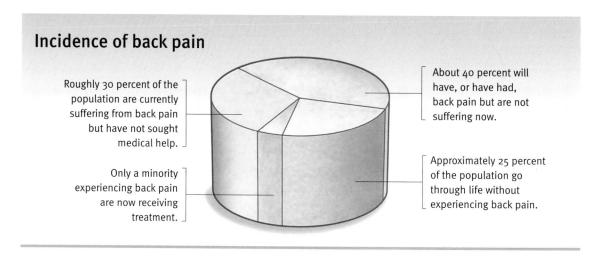

Incidence of back pain

Roughly 30 percent of the population are currently suffering from back pain but have not sought medical help.

Only a minority experiencing back pain are now receiving treatment.

About 40 percent will have, or have had, back pain but are not suffering now.

Approximately 25 percent of the population go through life without experiencing back pain.

Certain sports such as golf, bowling, and pitching in baseball – all of which can involve twisting and straining your back – lead to a higher incidence of back trouble. Competitive sports induce some people to train so intensively that they develop overuse injuries.

Abdominal muscles are often underused in everyday activities. If they are strong they help to support the spine by increasing pressure in the abdomen, which reduces stress on the lower spine. If your abdominal muscles are weak, your back will take more weight, making you prone to lower back pain.

The strength of back muscles, however, does not seem to affect the chances of having back trouble unless you are lifting particularly heavy weights. Most of us have back muscles that are adequate to cope with normal activities.

Inflexible hamstrings may predispose people to back pain. These muscles lengthen whenever you bend forward, so that your hips do most of the bending. If your hamstrings are stiff, your back has to bend further, and this will increase the risk of back problems. See pages 130–133 for exercises to stretch the hamstrings.

A stiff back may not cause trouble. However, therapies that aim to alleviate back pain through making the back more supple are often successful.

High-risk occupations

Many industrial surveys investigate back trouble among the work force, including workers with specific and very different tasks. In the construction industry, for example, the crane operator, the steel worker, and the unskilled laborer all belong to the same trade but experience widely differing loads on their spines. The evidence to date shows that workers who are required to lift heavy weights

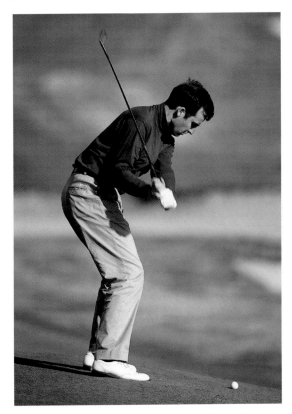

Strenuous sports
Golfers consistently twist their spines and expose themselves to a high incidence of back trouble.

manually are most at risk from back trouble. Unskilled and older laborers are most at risk – each year, about 22 percent of construction workers report back trouble, followed by nurses at 17 percent.

However, people such as office workers, who are engaged in sedentary jobs, are almost as much at risk as manual workers, particularly if the job entails driving long distances. For example, truck drivers, bus drivers, tractor drivers, and airplane pilots tend to develop lower back pain at an earlier age and show an increased X-ray evidence of degenerative disease in the spine. Vibration of the vehicles they drive and their position while driving may be factors.

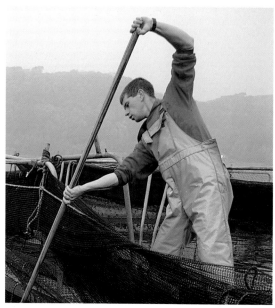

Hazardous job
Bending, twisting, and reaching movements can increase your chances of back trouble.

Hazardous activities

The following factors increase the chances of back problems. Often, the risks can be minimized by learning to lift and carry correctly, and by using appropriate equipment (*see Chapter 8*).

- Lifting weights manually.
- Lifting very heavy weights suddenly.
- Lifting an unexpectedly light weight.
- Bending, twisting, and reaching.
- Stooping and prolonged bending.
- Repetitive work with lighter loads.
- Static work postures – for example, driving, assembling electronic parts, sewing, weaving.
- Vibration – as in driving a tractor.
- Monotony and work dissatisfaction.
- Unacceptably high workloads (a maximum of half body weight for occasional handling, and of 40 percent of body weight for continuous lifting, was recommended as early as 1927).

- Rapid, repetitive handling tasks.
- Inappropriate working heights.
- Poor seating without backrest, arm supports, or swivel action.
- Inadequate space within which to turn or move.
- Poor viewing distance for sedentary workers.
- Tools/controls not within easy reach.

Psychological factors

No one can say for sure why some people are prone to back pain, while others who have a similar physique and live in similar circumstances are not. But the answer seems to lie partly in emotional or psychological factors.

We accept there are many examples of physical reactions governed by the emotions – blushing or fainting at the sight of blood – and it may well be that some people develop backache by similar mechanisms. On many occasions patients admit they have been under a lot of stress and ask, "Do you think it has anything to do with my back pain?" To me it seems no more than common sense to appreciate that continuous emotional or psychological stress can produce functional changes in the body, which influence the way you use your spine and muscles. Muscular tension resulting from suppressed emotions often causes neck pain and headaches as well as back pain.

Fluctuating moods

Day-to-day mood can affect the incidence of back trouble. Many people notice that on some days they can dig in the garden or do the housework without irritating their backs, while on other days their backs will ache at the slightest excuse.

Consider how often your posture reflects your mood. When you feel low and depressed your head tends to hang low and your shoulders will hunch.

If you feel resigned or defeated, you will probably slouch more. When you feel angry or irritable, you will be more careless as to how you use your back in bending and lifting.

Spend a few days observing how your mood affects your posture and how you use your back. Notice that when you feel buoyant, proud, and happy your back rarely acts up – at the very most you feel only an occasional twinge. Whenever there is psychological disharmony the chances are that there will also be physical dysfunction. As you become more aware of how your emotional state affects your posture, you may be able to avert back trouble by being extra careful and perhaps

resolving the inner conflict. It is all too easy for us to blame external circumstances, especially when we are suppressing anger and resentment. An awkward movement may just be "the straw that breaks the camel's back," while the emotional tension is the predisposing factor.

Stress: spinal and emotional

Back pain is the body's way of protesting against stress and enforcing a general slowing-down. Many people are under constant pressure for long periods, without adequate rest or vacations. They have lost touch with the needs of their bodies – the need for adequate physical recreation and for

Back pain at work

The incidence of back pain varies according to the kinds of occupation, which can be divided into three main categories – heavy, intermediate, and light. The sample occupations below are listed within each category in order of decreasing frequency of back trouble.

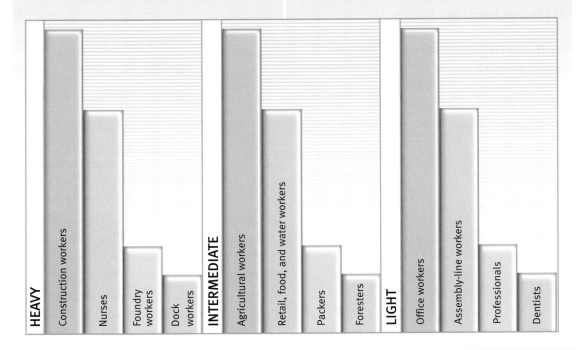

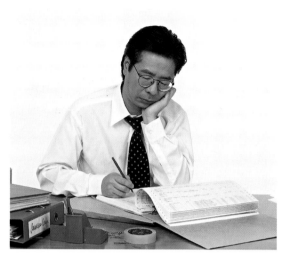

Risky posture
Leaning over a desk for long periods of time can put your spine under stress.

relaxation and sleep. I find that many business people who have developed acute back pain are under stress from high overheads, deadlines, jet travel, or simply striving to succeed in a highly competitive field. The 30- to 50-year-old man is at great risk and often he is driving himself mentally much harder than his emotional or physical system can manage.

My advice to such people is to take a few days off work, to reorder and balance their lives, and to reassess their priorities. This period allows them to increase their activity level gradually and follow any specific exercise.

Make your own diagnosis

There are many different causes of back pain. Almost any part of the spine can be damaged and cause pain. Disorders of other parts of the body, particularly the lungs, kidneys, and female reproductive organs, can also cause backache. Most back pain is neither severe nor serious, and can be treated adequately at home. However, since pain anywhere in the back can be a symptom of a serious disorder, it is important that you have some idea of what might be causing your pain, so that you can decide what action to take. Keep in mind that if your entire back is painful and other areas of your body ache and you have a fever, you probably have the flu, which is not covered in this book.

The charts on the following pages will help you to determine the cause of your pain, and will direct you to the sections in the book that are relevant to your disorder. Use whichever chart deals with the area of your pain, or with the part of your back that is most painful.

Answer the question at the top of the relevant chart with either "yes" or "no." Pain counts as "starting suddenly" if it builds up over no more than a few hours, perhaps overnight. You will be lead to your next question; progress through the chart until you reach a diagnosis box. This is just a very tentative diagnosis; only a doctor can give a firm diagnosis of your symptoms. It will, however, give you an idea of what might be causing your pain, and offer some advice on what you should do. If none of the diagnoses fit your symptoms, consult your doctor. Remember that symptoms vary greatly and these flow charts cover only the most common patterns of symptoms.

When the chart indicates you must seek urgent medical help, call your doctor or go to your nearest emergency department at once. When it suggests you should see your doctor, this is not an emergency, but you should see your doctor within a few days. When there is no advice to contact your doctor, see the appropriate section in the next chapter, which outlines the nature of various disorders, and gives more detailed advice on how you should cope. You may still, of course, want medical help, particularly if your pain is severe.

Lower back or leg pain

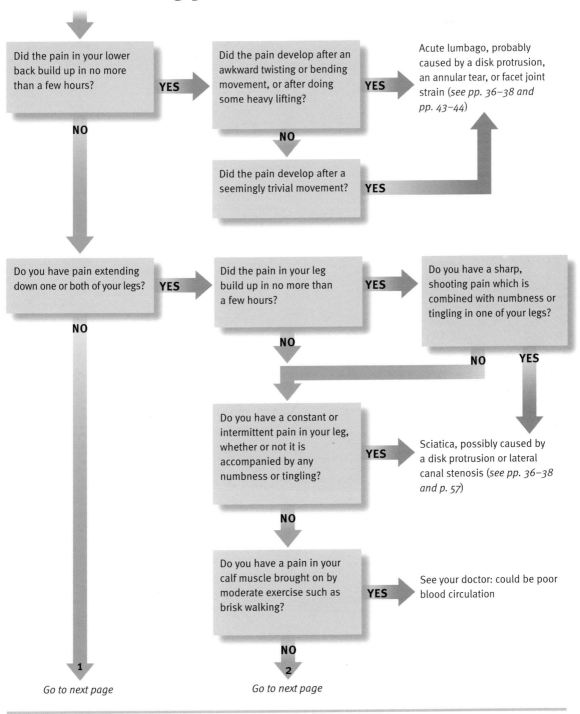

Did the pain in your lower back build up in no more than a few hours? — **YES** → **Did the pain develop after an awkward twisting or bending movement, or after doing some heavy lifting?** — **YES** → Acute lumbago, probably caused by a disk protrusion, an annular tear, or facet joint strain (*see pp. 36–38 and pp. 43–44*)

NO ↓

Did the pain develop after a seemingly trivial movement? — **YES** →

NO ↓

Do you have pain extending down one or both of your legs? — **YES** → **Did the pain in your leg build up in no more than a few hours?** — **YES** → **Do you have a sharp, shooting pain which is combined with numbness or tingling in one of your legs?**

NO ↓ (leg build up) **NO** ← → **YES**

Do you have a constant or intermittent pain in your leg, whether or not it is accompanied by any numbness or tingling? — **YES** → Sciatica, possibly caused by a disk protrusion or lateral canal stenosis (*see pp. 36–38 and p. 57*)

NO ↓

Do you have a pain in your calf muscle brought on by moderate exercise such as brisk walking? — **YES** → See your doctor: could be poor blood circulation

NO ↓

1
Go to next page

2
Go to next page

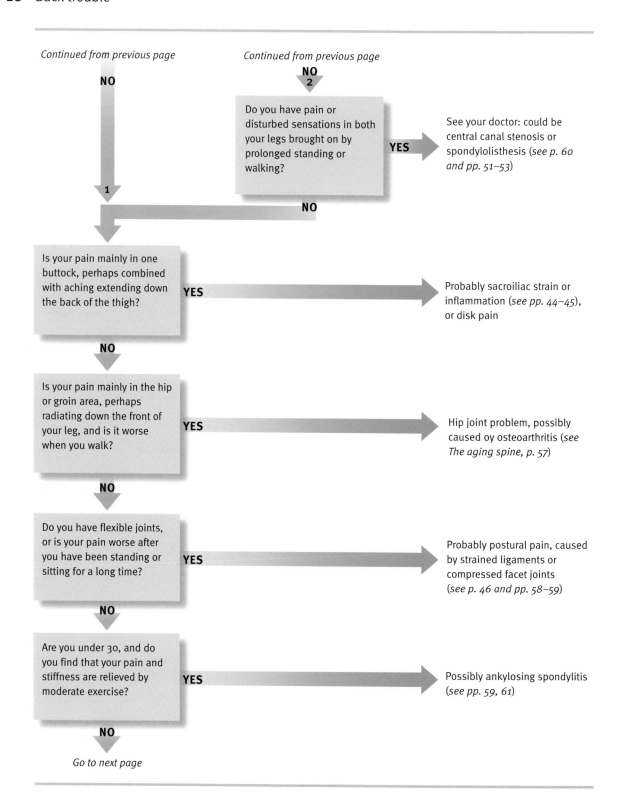

Continued from previous page

Continued from previous page

NO

NO
2

Do you have pain or disturbed sensations in both your legs brought on by prolonged standing or walking?

YES → See your doctor: could be central canal stenosis or spondylolisthesis (*see p. 60 and pp. 51–53*)

1

NO

Is your pain mainly in one buttock, perhaps combined with aching extending down the back of the thigh?

YES → Probably sacroiliac strain or inflammation (*see pp. 44–45*), or disk pain

NO

Is your pain mainly in the hip or groin area, perhaps radiating down the front of your leg, and is it worse when you walk?

YES → Hip joint problem, possibly caused oy osteoarthritis (*see The aging spine, p. 57*)

NO

Do you have flexible joints, or is your pain worse after you have been standing or sitting for a long time?

YES → Probably postural pain, caused by strained ligaments or compressed facet joints (*see p. 46 and pp. 58–59*)

NO

Are you under 30, and do you find that your pain and stiffness are relieved by moderate exercise?

YES → Possibly ankylosing spondylitis (*see pp. 59, 61*)

NO

Go to next page

Continued from previous page

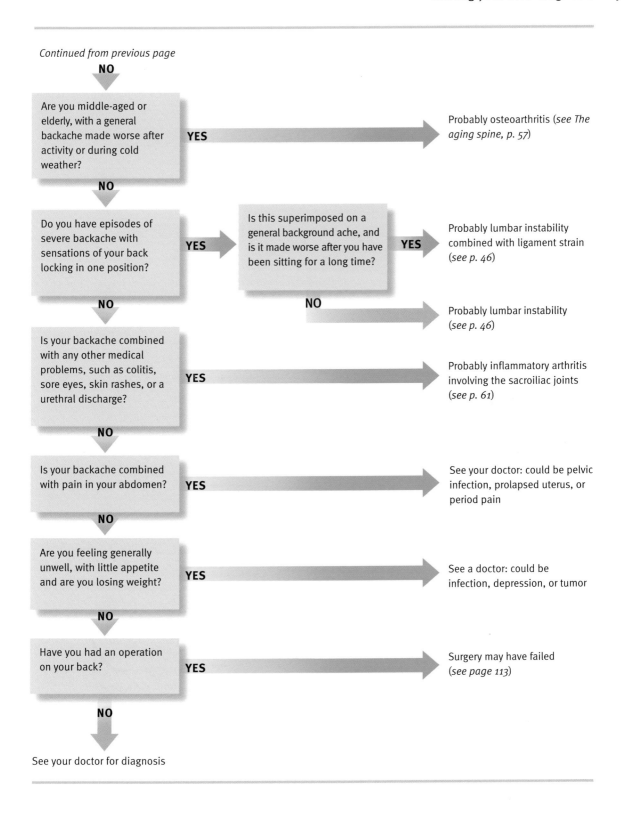

NO

Are you middle-aged or elderly, with a general backache made worse after activity or during cold weather?

YES → Probably osteoarthritis (*see The aging spine, p. 57*)

NO

Do you have episodes of severe backache with sensations of your back locking in one position?

YES → Is this superimposed on a general background ache, and is it made worse after you have been sitting for a long time?

YES → Probably lumbar instability combined with ligament strain (*see p. 46*)

NO → Probably lumbar instability (*see p. 46*)

NO

Is your backache combined with any other medical problems, such as colitis, sore eyes, skin rashes, or a urethral discharge?

YES → Probably inflammatory arthritis involving the sacroiliac joints (*see p. 61*)

NO

Is your backache combined with pain in your abdomen?

YES → See your doctor: could be pelvic infection, prolapsed uterus, or period pain

NO

Are you feeling generally unwell, with little appetite and are you losing weight?

YES → See a doctor: could be infection, depression, or tumor

NO

Have you had an operation on your back?

YES → Surgery may have failed (*see page 113*)

NO

See your doctor for diagnosis

Midback pain

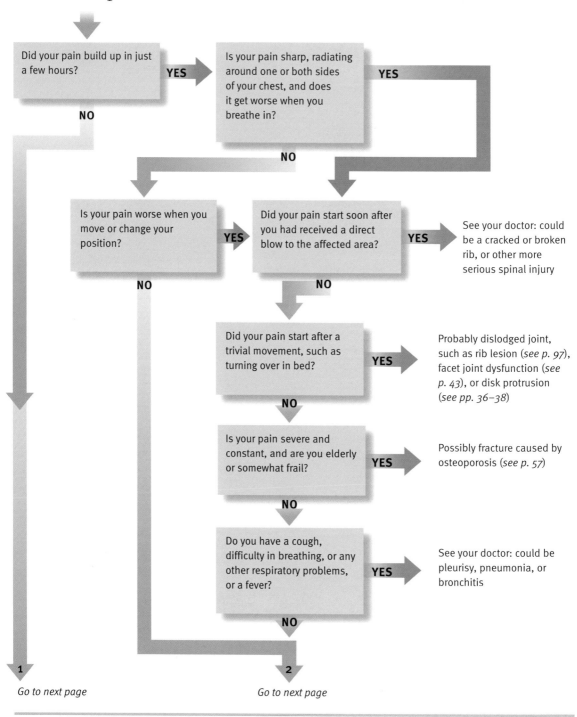

Did your pain build up in just a few hours?

YES → Is your pain sharp, radiating around one or both sides of your chest, and does it get worse when you breathe in?

NO

YES

NO

Is your pain worse when you move or change your position?

YES → Did your pain start soon after you had received a direct blow to the affected area?

YES → See your doctor: could be a cracked or broken rib, or other more serious spinal injury

NO

NO

Did your pain start after a trivial movement, such as turning over in bed?

YES → Probably dislodged joint, such as rib lesion (*see p. 97*), facet joint dysfunction (*see p. 43*), or disk protrusion (*see pp. 36–38*)

NO

Is your pain severe and constant, and are you elderly or somewhat frail?

YES → Possibly fracture caused by osteoporosis (*see p. 57*)

NO

Do you have a cough, difficulty in breathing, or any other respiratory problems, or a fever?

YES → See your doctor: could be pleurisy, pneumonia, or bronchitis

NO

1

Go to next page

2

Go to next page

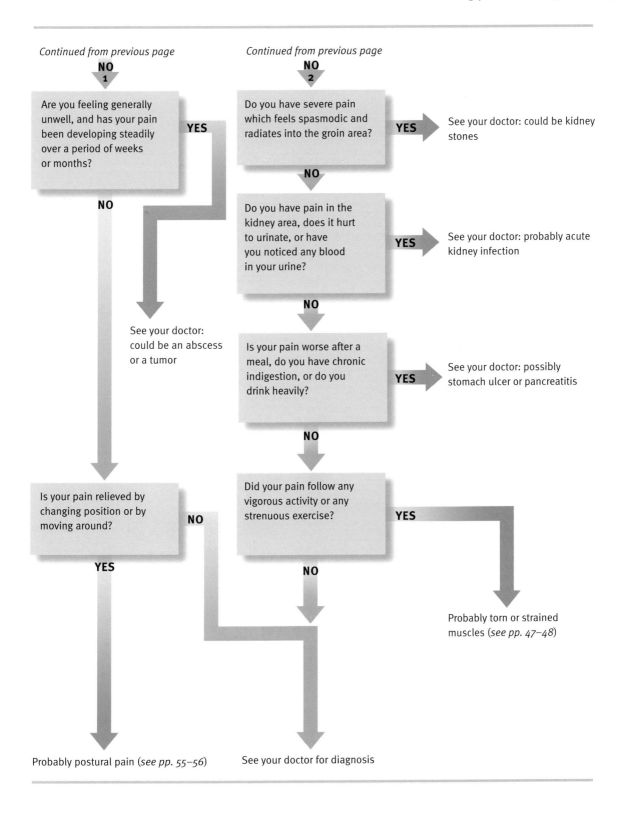

Continued from previous page
NO
1

Are you feeling generally unwell, and has your pain been developing steadily over a period of weeks or months?

YES

NO

Continued from previous page
NO
2

Do you have severe pain which feels spasmodic and radiates into the groin area?

YES → See your doctor: could be kidney stones

NO

Do you have pain in the kidney area, does it hurt to urinate, or have you noticed any blood in your urine?

YES → See your doctor: probably acute kidney infection

NO

See your doctor: could be an abscess or a tumor

Is your pain worse after a meal, do you have chronic indigestion, or do you drink heavily?

YES → See your doctor: possibly stomach ulcer or pancreatitis

NO

Is your pain relieved by changing position or by moving around?

NO

Did your pain follow any vigorous activity or any strenuous exercise?

YES

YES

NO

Probably torn or strained muscles (*see pp. 47–48*)

Probably postural pain (*see pp. 55–56*)

See your doctor for diagnosis

Neck, shoulder, or arm pain

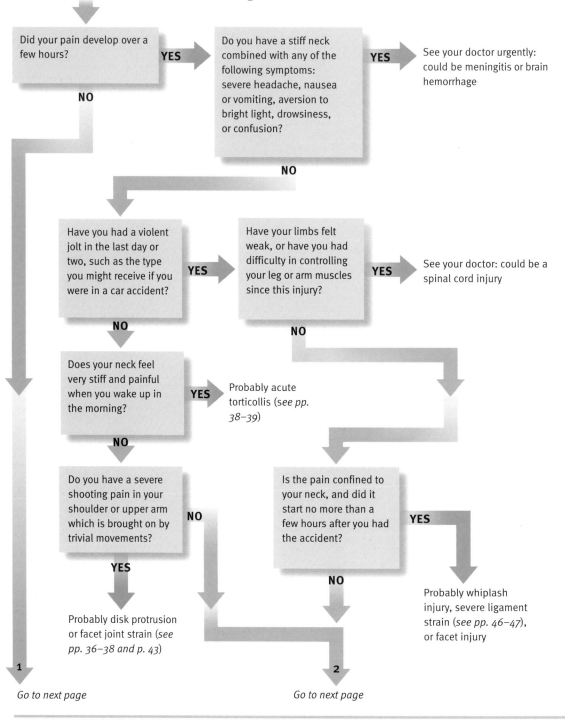

Did your pain develop over a few hours?

YES → Do you have a stiff neck combined with any of the following symptoms: severe headache, nausea or vomiting, aversion to bright light, drowsiness, or confusion?

YES → See your doctor urgently: could be meningitis or brain hemorrhage

NO

NO

Have you had a violent jolt in the last day or two, such as the type you might receive if you were in a car accident?

YES → Have your limbs felt weak, or have you had difficulty in controlling your leg or arm muscles since this injury?

YES → See your doctor: could be a spinal cord injury

NO

NO

Does your neck feel very stiff and painful when you wake up in the morning?

YES → Probably acute torticollis (*see pp. 38–39*)

NO

Do you have a severe shooting pain in your shoulder or upper arm which is brought on by trivial movements?

NO →

Is the pain confined to your neck, and did it start no more than a few hours after you had the accident?

YES →

YES ↓

NO

Probably disk protrusion or facet joint strain (*see pp. 36–38 and p. 43*)

Probably whiplash injury, severe ligament strain (*see pp. 46–47*), or facet injury

1

Go to next page

2

Go to next page

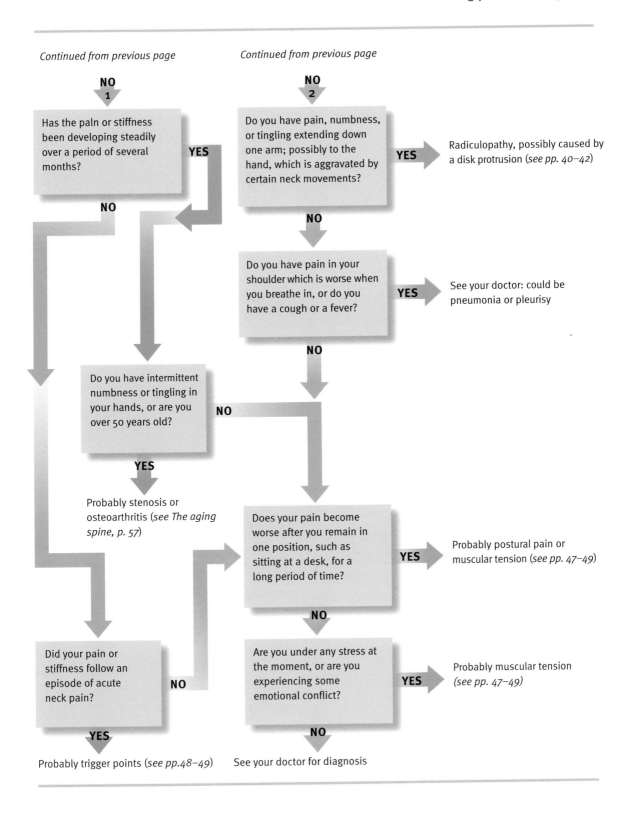

Continued from previous page

NO 1

Has the pain or stiffness been developing steadily over a period of several months?

YES

NO

Continued from previous page

NO 2

Do you have pain, numbness, or tingling extending down one arm; possibly to the hand, which is aggravated by certain neck movements?

YES → Radiculopathy, possibly caused by a disk protrusion (*see pp. 40–42*)

NO

Do you have pain in your shoulder which is worse when you breathe in, or do you have a cough or a fever?

YES → See your doctor: could be pneumonia or pleurisy

NO

Do you have intermittent numbness or tingling in your hands, or are you over 50 years old?

NO

YES

Probably stenosis or osteoarthritis (*see The aging spine, p. 57*)

Does your pain become worse after you remain in one position, such as sitting at a desk, for a long period of time?

YES → Probably postural pain or muscular tension (*see pp. 47–49*)

NO

Did your pain or stiffness follow an episode of acute neck pain?

NO

YES

Are you under any stress at the moment, or are you experiencing some emotional conflict?

YES → Probably muscular tension (*see pp. 47–49*)

NO

Probably trigger points (*see pp.48–49*)

See your doctor for diagnosis

3

Acute and Chronic Back Pain

The flow charts in the previous chapter will have given you a rough idea of the possible cause of your symptoms. However, diagnosing what has actually gone wrong, and which particular part of the back has been injured, can be extremely difficult, even for a specialist. If you have been overdoing things at home or at work and find yourself immobilized with pain, you might have strained a disk, torn a ligament or muscle, or strained several of the components of the back at once, but none of these show up on an ordinary X-ray.

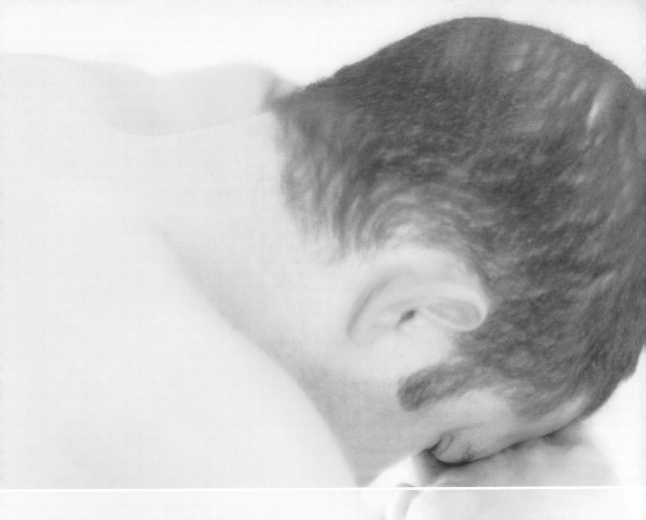

The healing process that follows a muscle or ligament injury is now more thoroughly understood than 50 years ago, when almost any pain resulting from a lower back injury would be described as "sciatica" or "lumbago," without any clear idea, in most cases, of what had gone wrong. Much research has focused on the disk – its functions, structure, and the way in which it ages. Almost all spinal problems are caused by mechanical strain or dysfunction – part of the structure is strained, stuck, or not functioning properly.

Disk problems

Although disks are very strong, they are vulnerable to twisting forces, which can rupture the outer layer of cartilage. This allows the pulpy gel inside to protrude, hence the term disk protrusion, or disk prolapse. Such a rupture can cause local pain by irritating the ligaments, the dural sheath and pain fibers in a disrupted annulus. Sometimes the disk presses on a nerve, causing severe pain down an arm or a leg. A disk becomes herniated when part of the nucleus completely detaches from the main nucleus, breaking through the posterior ligament. Disk problems are most common in the lower back, but they can also occur in the neck or, more rarely, in the middle back.

DISK PROTRUSIONS

These types of injuries are popularly known as "slipped disks," but this term is misleading because it suggests a disk has slipped out from between the vertebrae, somewhat like a loose washer. This is impossible since the disk is bound to the vertebrae by its fibrous outer layers. However, such a protrusion may cause pain at a distance from the damaged area, and little or no local pain. Such pain was once commonly called lumbago or lumbar sprain, terms used to describe any acute pain in the lower back, whatever the cause. However, medical opinion is divided as to whether this type of acute pain in the lower spine is generally caused by a disk protrusion or by an acute strain of one of the facet joints.

Disk problems are fairly common. The more severe protrusions generally affect young and middle-aged adults, because their disks contain a higher proportion of pulpy gel in the center than those of elderly people (*see p. 56*). Therefore, if the outer layers of a disk rupture in a young person, more gel can be extruded.

In the lower back

There may be little or no warning of an acute disk protrusion in the lower back. The pain tends to be of the deep, dull, aching kind, which may be felt in the middle of the lower back or to one side. It may radiate deep into the buttock, hip, or groin, with aching in your thighs, though these radiating pains may come and go.

Certain movements are painful and restricted. Bending forward hurts most though bending backward or to one side may be more painful.

Possible sites of pain

A disk protrusion usually causes severe pain around the immediate site and a dull ache may spread some distance. The pain may be central, or on one or both sides. For simplicity, these images show pain for the right-hand side.

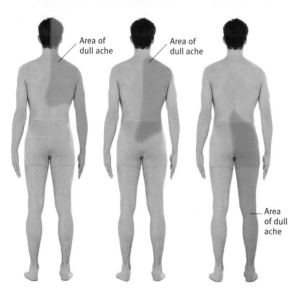

Area of dull ache

Area of dull ache

Area of dull ache

Protrusion in the neck

Protrusion in the midback

Protrusion in the lower back

Types of disk protrusion

A damaged disk can protrude in several ways, but it doesn't have to be painful. Symptoms depend on the nature of the damage, the amount of nucleus that protrudes, and the surface it presses against. Ruptures in the annulus fibrosus can cause painful lesions. When the nucleus has protruded far enough to press against the ligament, dura, or nerve it is also painful. As the disk degenerates with age, small splits frequently occur in the layers of the annulus fibrosus, but these changes are often painless.

End-plate lesions

The outer layers are undamaged but the end plates of the vertebrae have given way. The inner gel is still contained within the annulus fibrosus.

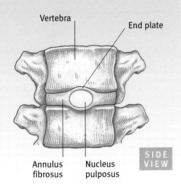

Vertebra

End plate

Annulus fibrosus

Nucleus pulposus

SIDE VIEW

Degenerative changes

The disk is internally fissured, but the nucleus does not stream into the ruptured annulus fibrosus.

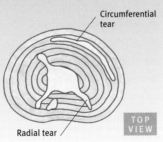

Circumferential tear

Radial tear

TOP VIEW

The annulus fibrosus is ruptured and the nucleus begins to leak through the small splits.

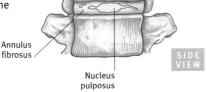

Annulus fibrosus

Nucleus pulposus

SIDE VIEW

Disk lesions

The prolapsed disk protrudes far enough to press against the posterior ligament.

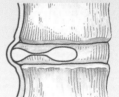

Ligament

SIDE VIEW

Part of the nucleus has become detached, and bursts through the annulus fibrosus to press against the ligament.

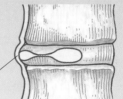

SIDE VIEW

The protruding disk has ruptured the ligament.

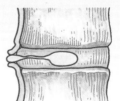

SIDE VIEW

The nucleus leaks out through the ruptured annulus fibrosus and posterior ligament.

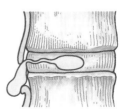

SIDE VIEW

You may lean to one side or find you are unable to straighten up fully. Quite often, the pain increases suddenly when you cough, laugh, sneeze, or strain. Usually, if you try to walk around, the pain builds up in intensity, particularly if you attempt further bending or reaching movements.

Prolonged sitting may offer a temporary relief, but when you try to stand up again the pain and restriction may be even greater. On the other hand, sitting may be excruciatingly painful, depending on how the affected disk is protruding. Often, the pain is continuous but it can be partly or completely relieved if you lie flat (though not necessarily on your back).

The disk protrusion may or may not resolve (reduce in size) spontaneously in a few days or it may take weeks or months. Improvement of symptoms depends partly on the size and position of the protrusion but also on your response to the pain: if your muscles tense up, you will find it increasingly difficult to become mobile again, so delaying your recovery. If the pain is so severe you can barely move, modify your activities temporarily, perhaps by lying down for two or three days, but keep as mobile as you can.

Some treatments may speed your recovery – mobilizing exercises, manipulation to reduce pain and improve mobility, and trigger point needling (*see p. 158*) to reduce pain and to relax muscles.

In the midback

Disk protrusions in the midback are less common because the region is less mobile and the disks are smaller. If they cause symptoms of pressure on the spinal cord they may need surgery.

In the neck

Typically, you wake in the morning and cannot lift your head from the pillow; turning your head is extremely painful and difficult. Usually, it is equally difficult to bend your head backward or forward. The condition is often called torticollis, or wry neck. The restricted movement is typically caused by a physical derangement rather than a disease. The term can also apply to facet joint strain (*see p. 43*), and some experts still regard it as a form of muscle spasm.

Normally, you feel better within five to ten days without any particular treatment. Recovery can be hastened by gentle traction from a manipulative

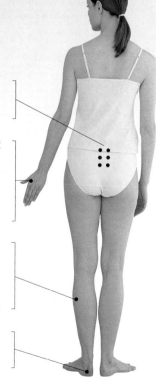

Acupuncture for lumbago

An acupuncturist (*see p. 160*) will select certain points on different energy channels, or meridians, to help treat lumbago.

Local points on the bladder meridian are often chosen.

A large intestine point on the hand may be treated – digestion problems may be linked to a displaced vertebra.

This point on the gallbladder meridian is influential in treating damaged muscles and tendons.

For sedation and pain relief, a point on the foot may be chosen.

Causes of disk protrusion

Most painful disk protrusions develop from nonpainful ones. As this illustration shows, an awkward twisting or bending movement compresses the damaged disk first on one side, then suddenly on the other, causing pain.

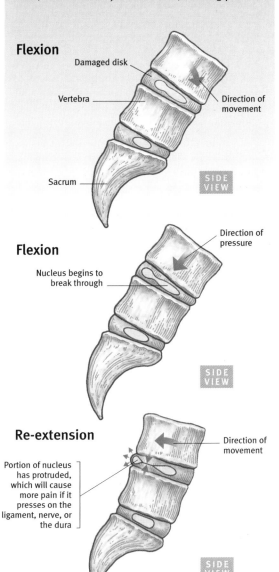

Flexion

Damaged disk

Vertebra

Direction of movement

Sacrum

SIDE VIEW

Flexion

Direction of pressure

Nucleus begins to break through

SIDE VIEW

Re-extension

Direction of movement

Portion of nucleus has protruded, which will cause more pain if it presses on the ligament, nerve, or the dura

SIDE VIEW

therapist, by wearing a soft collar at night to prevent further strain, by acupuncture to relieve muscle tension, and by mobilizing exercises. Although torticollis is painful and unpleasant, you should be able to continue normal activities.

Torticollis can occasionally occur in young children, when it may be caused by a throat or ear infection. Elderly or late middle-aged people rarely suffer from acute torticollis: the symptoms at this age tend to become chronic and are part of the general process of degeneration.

CHRONIC DISK PROBLEMS

Most acute disk episodes get better as the swelling and inflammation settle. This may take weeks or months. However, 10 to 30 percent continue to cause problems for longer.

In the lower back

Problems in the lumbar spine will probably cause aching and stiffness after sitting down. You may also feel sharp twinges and occasionally your back might "lock" in one position. The pain is usually located on one side of the back and you may also have some intermittent leg pain, possibly with pins and needles. These symptoms, combined with a background of dull aching, are common in middle-aged back sufferers and may often be provoked by postural strains or excessive lifting and bending.

Your long-term outlook is quite good because, as you progress into late middle age or old age, the spine stiffens and the ligaments ossify, making the overall structure much more stable. Until then, you may get relief with therapies such as manipulation, exercise rehabilitation, and prolotherapy (*see p. 101*). Few people need surgery. Above all, exercise regularly to strengthen the support of the spine, improve your posture, stay as active as you can, and avoid sports or activities that put your back at risk.

In the neck

If you have two or three episodes of acute neck pain early in adult life, you may develop frequent deep aching in the shoulder and upper back as you approach middle age.

Every now and again you may experience a milder version of the stiff and painful neck. You might notice grinding and crunching noises on sudden movements of the head and neck. This is due to thinning of the disks combined with greater compression strain on the small joints at the back of the neck and strained ligaments.

Once a disk thins, the ligaments slacken and can no longer fulfill their stabilizing function, thus making that whole segment of the spine less stable. You may get intermittent nerve root pain, perhaps with pins and needles in one or both hands, as the nerve roots are temporarily compressed.

Treatment for the neck is similar to that for the lower spine, though you are more likely to develop patterns of chronic muscular tension in the neck area. Try relaxation (*see p. 68*) to prevent this.

COMPRESSED NERVES

Sometimes, when a disk bulges to one side, it presses on a nerve root that exits from the spinal column. You feel pain in the immediate area and wherever the nerve leads to, usually the leg or arm on that side. A pinched nerve can cause other disturbances of sensation, such as numbness or pins and needles. If this persists, the nerve root can be damaged, weakening the muscles controlled by that nerve. The sheath containing the nerve can inflame as a reaction to being pinched.

Lumbar radiculopathy (sciatica)

If a disk in your lower back presses on the lumbar nerve roots, you will feel pain down one leg (commonly called sciatica), perhaps with numbness or tingling in a small area of the leg or foot. In more severe cases, when the nerve has been damaged, certain muscle groups in the leg may be weakened. Although the problem of sciatica usually starts with back pain, after a few days the pain decreases in the back but becomes correspondingly severe in the leg.

In some cases of sciatica, the pain is severe and unrelenting, no matter what position you adopt. However, the pain may subside with short intervals of rest. Fortunately, most disk protrusions resolve themselves spontaneously. After a while, the pain in your leg will ease, and the tingling will gradually disappear. You might, however, be left with a small patch of numbness in your foot, and perhaps some residual weakness when you try pulling up your foot or your big toe.

About 90 percent of severe cases of sciatica clear up within three months, but if there is no improvement after two weeks, consult your doctor. Manipulation, traction, acupuncture, careful posture, and exercises can be tried but are usually not as successful as injections. A minority may eventually need surgery.

Cervical radiculopathy (brachialgia)

The pain can be caused by a protruding cervical disk bulging sideways and pressing on a nerve root, or causing inflammation, as it exits from the spinal canal. This will cause severe pain in your arm or hand, according to which nerve is compressed. It may be accompanied by pins and needles or a patch of numbness.

If the nerve root is damaged, causing weakness or loss of muscular reflex, your pain may be severe and will not settle easily with rest, manipulation, or acupuncture. If this is the case, you may be given a collar – although prolonged wear is not advisable – or an injection.

Nerves to the hands and feet

The lumbar nerve roots, that make up the sciatic nerve, leave the spinal canal between the fourth lumbar and second sacral vertebrae and run to the feet. A pinched sciatic nerve sends a sharp, shooting pain down one leg, perhaps with numbness or pins and needles. The cervical nerves leave the canal at the base of the neck and run to the hands. The femoral nerve's lumbar roots leave between the second and fifth lumbar vertebra.

Compressed nerve

The nucleus of the disk protrudes between the vertebrae and pinches a nerve as it leaves the spinal canal. Pain can occur in all areas supplied by the nerve.

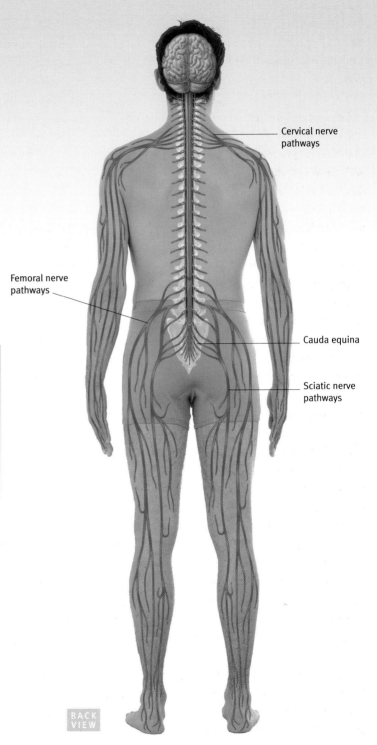

Cervical nerve pathways

Femoral nerve pathways

Cauda equina

Sciatic nerve pathways

BACK VIEW

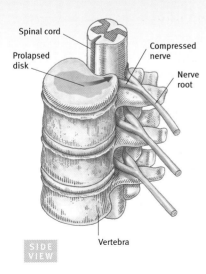

Spinal cord

Prolapsed disk

Compressed nerve

Nerve root

Vertebra

SIDE VIEW

CHRONIC LUMBAR AND CERVICAL RADICULOPATHY

Prolonged lumbar or cervical radiculopathy pain may be caused by a continuing disk protrusion, epidural root fibrosis, or lateral canal stenosis (*see p. 57*). Rarely, chronic cervical radiculopathy may occur when the cervical nerves are trapped between the collar bone and the first rib by an extra rib (cervical rib), by a tumor at the base of the neck or by tight scalene muscles in the neck.

Continuing disk protrusion

In a few cases of lumbar or cervical radiculopathy, the disk prolapse does not resolve but continues to press on the nerve. If your pain continues after eight weeks of conservative treatment, see a back specialist who may order a scan to find out which disk is prolapsed.

Depending on the degree of pain, the extent of nerve damage, and your general disability, he may recommend an operation to remove the protruding part of the disk. Occasionally, a piece of disk cartilage can become completely detached and lie wedged against the nerve. Once diagnosed, the fragment can be removed by surgery.

Chronic lumbar radiculopathy, from whatever cause, can leave you in severe pain for a long period and you need strategies for coping with it (*see Chapter 9*). Manipulation, acupuncture, traction, or rest rarely have any lasting benefit. Spinal injections may bring relief. Though it may take six to nine months, disk prolapse is more likely to resolve spontaneously.

Epidural root fibrosis

After disk prolapse or surgery, the nerve root sleeve may become scarred with fibrous tissue and adhere to the walls of the spinal canal. Pain is provoked when you bend over, stride out, or increase any

Epidural root fibrosis

Inflexible scar tissue growing on the injured dural root sleeve can become attached to the bony walls of the spinal canal, trapping the nerve root. This makes any bending movements, which pull on the nerve, very painful.

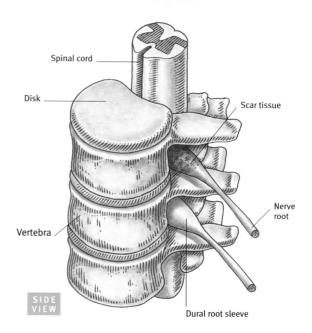

Spinal cord

Disk

Scar tissue

Nerve root

Vertebra

SIDE VIEW

Dural root sleeve

upright activity. Usually, the pain is relieved by straightening up or by lying down flat, although it may linger for hours.

As the months go by your range of motion does not increase since the scar tissue is firm. If the root does not become free you may need exercises to stretch the fibrous tissue little by little. There are no treatments with proven success for this problem. Experimental treatments include injections of cortisone, or of enzymes to break down the scar tissue, and dissection of scar tissue adhesions via a scope (epiduroscopy).

Joint strain and dysfunction

If a joint is twisted or jerked, causing severe pain as the ligaments and joint capsule are irritated, it may "stick" or lock up. In medical terms, this is a strain; when the "stuck" position is maintained by local muscle spasms, it is a dysfunction.

FACET JOINTS

Acute back pain is often caused when one of the small facet joints that link the vertebrae together is strained or jammed. Such a problem can occur at any level of the spine, but, as with disk trouble, it is more likely to affect the neck and lower back. The pain comes from irritation of the facet joints, and is often described as mechanical back pain.

In the lower back

An awkward twisting or bending movement may injure the ligaments, muscles, and capsule of a facet joint. In a middle-aged person, when the disks have started to degenerate and the ligaments may be slack, the facet joints may experience more continuous strain.

The symptoms are similar to those caused by a protruding disk in the lower back, since the pain may be very severe and restrict your movements for the first two or three days. Pain may radiate to your buttock, hip, lower abdomen, and thighs but, unlike a disk protrusion, without a sharp pain down the leg or any numbness or weakness.

This type of problem responds to brief rest, pain medication, exercise, and manipulation. As in cases of minor disk protrusion, much depends on your health and fitness. If you have good muscle tone and can relax properly, you will probably recover more quickly than someone with slack muscles or someone who tenses up in response to pain.

Facet joint dysfunction

A joint is stuck or jammed if the facets have trapped a small piece or fold of the capsule between them.

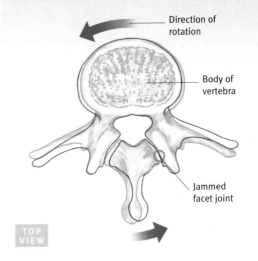

Direction of rotation

Body of vertebra

Jammed facet joint

TOP VIEW

A rotation strain
The facet joint is strained when the spine is rotated, often at the same time as bending or straightening up.

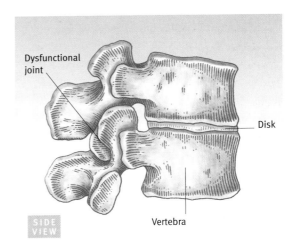

Dysfunctional joint

Disk

SIDE VIEW

Vertebra

Dysfunctional joint
If the bones slip slightly out of line but still overlap the joint becomes dysfunctional.

In the midback

Awkward twisting or bending strains may also set up acute midback pain, radiating like a girdle around the side and even to the front of the chest or upper abdomen. Initially, it can be so severe that it is painful even to breathe.

The same set of causes may be involved here as in other spinal problems; for example, if you don't warm up before playing sports or if you are lifting furniture. Simply turning over in bed at night or sleeping awkwardly can cause it. Even after the initial pain and restriction have eased, many people feel some residual pain. Movements continue to be limited for weeks, months, or even years, unless they receive adequate treatment, which generally entails manipulation.

Less severe midback pain is relatively common and may occur at almost any age, though it more often affects young and middle-aged adults. You usually feel better if you adopt a suitable position, but will soon be reminded of it when you try to change position or turn in a particular direction. This type of pain is variously caused by the facet joints, muscle trigger points (see p. 48), or rib lesions, when the joints between the ribs and the thoracic vertebrae become jammed or stuck.

In the neck

Problems involving any of the joints in the neck will make it stiff and painful. This condition has very similar symptoms to a disk protrusion in the neck, and the term torticollis can apply to both types of problem. If you have a facet joint strain in the neck, it will be painful and your movements will be limited in certain directions when you turn or bend your head to one side.

Most people prefer to lie down, taking the weight of the head off the neck, but others find this makes it even worse. The solution is to keep the neck straight and support it: at night, try a soft collar or a rolled and twisted towel around your neck to stop your head from lolling from side to side when you sleep. This eases the pain and aids the healing process.

These episodes rarely lead to any long-term problems, but sometimes, after weeks or even months, pain may persist, together with restricted movement and aching extending into the shoulder-blade region. Trigger point areas may develop (see p. 48), but on the whole manipulation or injection of the joint is extremely useful.

SACROILIAC JOINT STRAIN

This most commonly occurs in young to middle-aged women; men, especially athletes, may also suffer. The reason why this injury is more common among women is probably because the tough fibrous ligament of the sacroiliac joint (see right) tends to relax during pregnancy in preparation for childbirth. The initial cause of a sacroiliac strain may be a twisting or bending movement. You will probably know when the pain started and which movement was the one that caused it. It may occur, for example, when you unexpectedly step off a curb – your muscles are unprepared for the strain and the ligaments absorb the force.

Once the sacroiliac joint is strained or stuck, you will feel a sharp pain in the upper inner area of the buttock when you put your foot down or strike the heel on that side. There will also be a background, wedge-shaped area of pain, radiating deep into the lower buttock. If the pain is severe, it may travel farther down the back of the thigh. Pain from the sacroiliac joint may be referred to the groin and/or the outer thigh. In general, this problem does not cause very severe pain. It can, however, be a nagging nuisance that aches even when you are trying to rest. Many of these acute joint strains will

Sacroiliac joint

The fused spinal segments which make up the sacrum have two crescent-shaped surfaces, one on each side. These are the articular surfaces of the sacrum. They fit snugly into two corresponding surfaces, one on each iliac bone. Together, the two iliac bones and the sacrum make up the pelvic girdle. The female pelvis is shown in the illustration below; the male pelvis is slightly narrower and deeper. The ball of each thigh bone fits into the socket on each iliac bone.

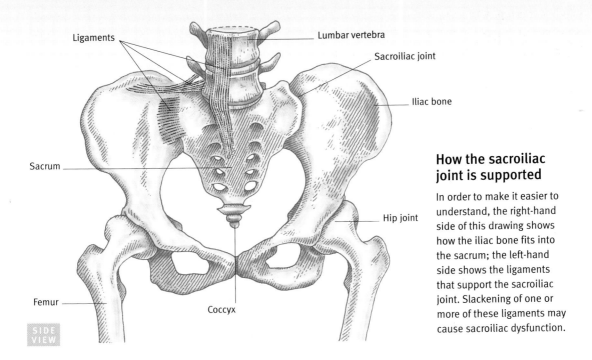

Ligaments

Lumbar vertebra

Sacroiliac joint

Iliac bone

Sacrum

Hip joint

Femur

Coccyx

SIDE VIEW

How the sacroiliac joint is supported

In order to make it easier to understand, the right-hand side of this drawing shows how the iliac bone fits into the sacrum; the left-hand side shows the ligaments that support the sacroiliac joint. Slackening of one or more of these ligaments may cause sacroiliac dysfunction.

settle down spontaneously within a week or two, but if they persist they will generally respond quickly to manipulation. However, if the ligament has been strained more than once or twice, you are likely to feel long-term twinges or aches accompanied by occasional flare-ups. There are effective ways of tightening the ligaments with sclerosant injections (*see p. 101*), in order to hold the joint more firmly. If the symptoms last more than a month, see your doctor: you may have a chronic inflammation rather than just a sprained joint. Injections of steroids may be helpful.

Ligament injuries

An acute attack of back pain is unlikely to be due entirely to strained ligaments. However, there are certain types of injury in which ligaments may be the main cause of pain. Ligaments can take longer to heal than a fractured bone. Indeed, they often fail to heal completely, being overstretched or restricted by adhesions (matted fibrous tissue which prevents the ligaments from gliding over the surface of the bone). This can become a source of chronic pain.

Slack or strained ligaments

As you age, the disks become thinner and the vertebrae move closer together. The ligaments that once supported the spine firmly will slacken, so the joints are looser. Ligaments become slack during pregnancy, and an injury to the spine can also strain joints. Once this happens, the facet joints are likely to become strained from time to time. It is all somewhat like a worn machine with a loose drive belt or pulley: any undue strain will probably throw something out of gear.

Minor strains and changes of position cause a feeling of the back "going out," or locking. This results in a sharp pain combined with a deep, diffuse ache. Frequent locking episodes in the neck or the lower back create a sense of instability. The sensation comes from the facet or sacroiliac joints being stuck. If the disk is also involved, prolonged bending or stooping activities will cause pain and stiffness, and you may be unable to straighten up. Your lifestyle is likely to be affected: gardening and DIY jobs can become a problem.

If your ligaments are also strained or weak, you will feel pain after prolonged sitting and inactivity, and a change of position will tend to set off acute twinges. Ligaments are weakest at the ends, where they are attached to the bone, and this is where they can be overstretched. They will then become inflamed and cause a background ache much of the time. This pain will probably be most severe first thing in the morning, but will wear off when you move around. It is aggravated by vigorous exercise or activity, but also increases if you sit still for a long time.

This type of back pain is difficult to cope with since you never seem to be entirely free of trouble. The response to treatment is variable, but attention to your posture, general fitness, and good muscle tone, as well as exercises, can help.

Each acute episode can be treated with modified activities, manipulation, exercises, or acupuncture. If you have frequent attacks of pain, you will know what works best for you. Lasting effects can be achieved by stabilizing the "unstable" segments, with exercise or prolotherapy (*see p. 101*), for example. Spinal fusion is reserved for those with more severe mechanical instability.

As you become older, your spine usually becomes more stable again because your ligaments will tend to harden, and the whole structure becomes stiffer.

Whiplash syndrome

If the neck is bent violently backward or forward – for example, in a rear-end collision – the ligaments surrounding the joints in the neck are strained or, rarely, ruptured. Because the muscles are not poised to absorb the shock, the joints are forced to the extreme of their range. Since this is limited by the ligaments, these absorb the impact. Such an accident may also damage the disks, muscles, and facet joints in the neck. The resulting symptoms are commonly called "whiplash syndrome."

Many cases of whiplash syndrome initially pass unnoticed, because an X-ray will not reveal the strain of the ligaments, and internal bleeding may be very slow. However, over a number of hours, perhaps overnight, the neck will become very stiff and painful.

It is important to manage whiplash syndrome in its early stages, because otherwise it can create long-term problems. If there is any likelihood that you have suffered a whiplash injury, consult your doctor, who should prescribe simple pain medication and advise you to keep active and to avoid wearing a collar. The best early treatment is manual traction given by a physical therapist as well as range-of-motion exercises (*see Chapter 7*) and postural advice (*see Chapter 8*).

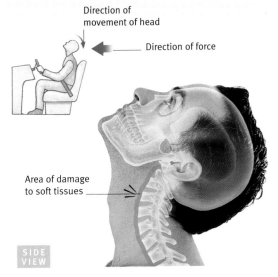

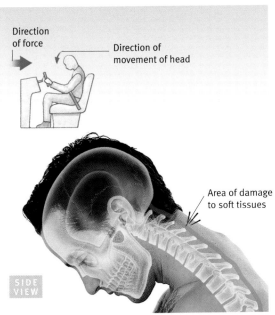

Muscular strains

Injuries to the muscles in the back and neck are not as common as most people imagine. Many painful conditions of the back are often described by doctors as "muscular" or "ligamentous." To some extent this description may be true, since the muscles and ligaments are part and parcel of the workings of the back and can be affected by undue tension and associated strain. Tense muscles may be incidental to a disk protrusion or facet joint strain.

A purely muscular injury to the back typically happens to an athlete undertaking vigorous exercise after insufficient stretching and warming up. The pain will probably start quite suddenly, and will recur after repetition of the action that initially triggered it. Reaching or pulling movements are likely to aggravate it, and the muscles might be tender and slightly swollen. There may be some internal bleeding if the muscle is injured.

Muscular strains can be a nuisance, but they usually respond to brief rest and physical therapy. Few such injuries take more than two weeks to heal.

Chronic muscular tension

Occasionally, muscles become chronically tense and cause myofascial pain. This is usually a result of poor posture, and is common among people who spend long hours leaning over a desk or table, or factory workers who stand or sit for long periods with their arms outstretched as their hands manipulate small objects.

If your work involves such a posture, it is very important to ensure that your desk or work surface and your chair are the right height for you (*see p. 143*). If you are tall, you will have to droop your head and shoulders a little further to reach a working height designed for an average-sized person. This may put greater strain on the muscles which are constantly working to support the load. Tense muscles may be relaxed through massage or exercises to stretch them (*see Chapter 7*).

If your work involves constantly repeating a pattern of movements in the arms and shoulders – for instance, working on a production line – your muscles become tired. When this happens, the vulnerable trigger point areas (*see opposite*) may tighten up and start referring pain to other areas. This is slightly different from the static postural pain that a draftsman can develop poring over his drawings, but both are tests of endurance for the muscle groups, one through repetitive action and the other through sustained position.

Psychological stress is a factor in determining which individual performing the same activities in the same place of work is most susceptible to developing chronic neck pain, shoulder pain, or headaches. A high level of anxiety and frustration can cause increased muscular tension, particularly in the neck. If you are unable to release these tensions, either vocally or through some physical outlet, you might suppress your emotions by tensing your muscles.

Most people who develop neck pain will ask at some time or other: "Is it because of the draft I was in from that open window in the car or the cold corridor I was standing in for an hour or two last night?" There is an element of truth in this – cold drafts or winds, by rapidly cooling the skin and superficial muscles, cause increased muscular tension, which reduces the blood flow. Together, these factors can contribute to the development of trigger points.

Beverages such as coffee, which stimulate the nervous system, can cause increased excitability of the muscles, which in turn makes them more likely to contract over a period of time. Excessive alcohol fatigues your muscles, and over a long period it can even damage the muscle cells. It has also been recognized that, in susceptible people, certain foods can cause abnormal reactions involving the muscles, producing widespread aching. Unless you are aware of this possibility, it may very well remain an undetected cause of your back pain.

Trigger points

Pain from spinal structures can radiate outward to surrounding areas and set up secondary points of tension, which become taut little bands or knots in the muscle. This used to be called fibrositis but is now referred to as trigger point phenomena or, somewhat dauntingly, myofascial dysfunction. It is very common in the neck and shoulders of people who are under postural stress or experiencing an acute episode of neck pain.

There are various recognized common positions at which these trigger points develop, and if you touch one, you will feel a tense, hard nodule which may twitch as a response to deep pressure and spread pain into whichever area of the shoulder, arm or chest is already hurting.

This problem must be approached in several ways. In the first place, a dysfunction of a spinal joint must be corrected. If this is not the primary cause of the pain, the tender points of the muscle need to be relaxed with massage, physical therapy, or passive stretching exercises, a local injection or dry needling (a form of acupuncture called intramuscular stimulation).

You must alter your circumstances at work or at home to prevent tension and pain from returning. Improve your seating, adapt tasks so your back is under less strain, and alter the height of work surfaces. Ergonomic design – adapting an environment to suit the person working in it – is a very important factor in eliminating back or neck pain due to poor posture (*see Chapter 8*).

Trigger points

There are several common sites of pain caused by muscle trigger points. These are some of the most common. The specific trigger points are indicated on the figures as black crosses. The dark red tints are the main areas of referred pain; the lighter tints show the maximum extent of referred pain.

Face and neck

Shoulders and neck

Key

Trigger points   X
Referred pain   ▪

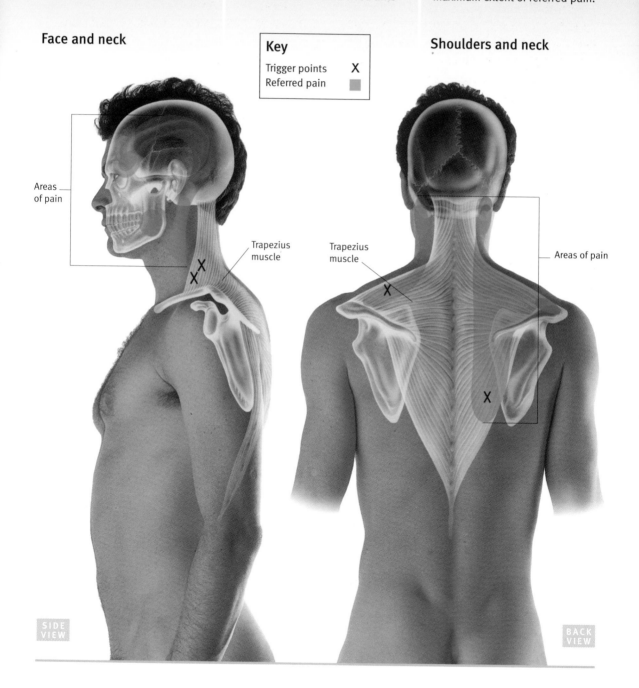

Areas of pain

Trapezius muscle

Trapezius muscle

Areas of pain

SIDE VIEW

BACK VIEW

Injuries to the spine

If you fall from a height or are struck on the spine by a heavy object – even if you can get up and move around – make sure you consult a doctor, since there is a risk of paralysis.

The three main types of minor fracture are shown below. In avulsion, the tip of the transverse or spinous process is cracked or pulled off. A violent muscular action can cause this, so athletes are typical victims. You feel a sudden and severe pain at first. Refrain from any activity that provokes the pain until the injury is healed.

A microfracture can occur without a violent injury – for example, just by lifting a heavy weight. The best treatment is to modify your activity. Most heal spontaneously but people with continuing back trouble may have one that has failed to unite.

Compression fractures occur when a vertebra collapses entirely. A common sufferer is the elderly person who has considerable thinning of the bones (*see Osteoporosis, p. 57*). If you are elderly and you feel a sudden, severe, and immobilizing back pain (usually in the mid or lower back) without any particular external injury, consult your doctor. You may have a visible bump and hunch forward. Initially, treatment is pain medication, rest, and bracing but later on you may be given drug therapy (*see p. 101*) to encourage the bone to remineralize. However, once the wedge compression has formed, the resulting hunch is likely to remain.

The best way of tackling osteoporosis is to prevent it entirely by staying active into old age, and have an adequate intake of calcium and vitamin D, since this encourages the continued renewal of the stronger components of the bone structure.

Minor fractures

Violent injury to the spine may result in the fracture of a vertebra and consequent damage to the spinal cord. However, many less serious fractures can be caused by quite a trivial movement.

Minor fractures, which are unlikely to involve damage to the spinal cord but can cause problems nevertheless, fall into three main categories – avulsion, microfractures, and compression fractures.

Avulsion

One of the processes may be cracked, or the tip of one can be torn off. This injury is usually caused by violent overuse of the muscle attached to the process.

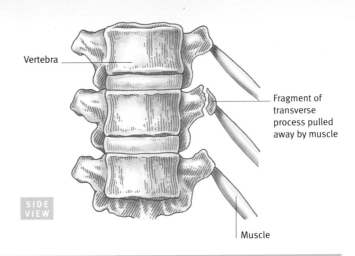

Vertebra

Fragment of transverse process pulled away by muscle

SIDE VIEW

Muscle

A fourth type of minor fracture, stress fractures can occur in the lower back if you put a lot of stress on the spine – for example, in vigorous physical training, athletics, and gymnastics. Stress fractures may gradually develop in young athletes who train excessively. Initially, there is a localized ache or pain during activity which eases when you stop. Gradually, the pain comes on earlier, is more severe, and lasts longer after the activity. Eventually, it interferes with any running, jumping, or jarring activities – even walking or standing.

Occasionally, this stress reaction can fracture through the arch (*see Spondylolysis, p. 52*). Such acute stress fractures are best diagnosed with a CT or bone scan (*see pp. 80–81*). You should avoid any aggravating activities for up to six months but try to keep fit in other ways and strengthen your stabilizing muscles.

Coccydynia is a minor fracture that occurs when you fall on to the coccyx, or tailbone. A persistent painful bruising stops you from sitting comfortably. Normally, it heals on its own, but if the pain stays severe after several months, a local injection can reduce inflammation. A minority need surgery.

Spondylolysis and spondylolisthesis

Vertebrae in the lower back occasionally slip out of line significantly, causing back pain if the joints or ligaments are irritated. Nerves may be trapped, producing leg pain, numbness, or pins and needles in the legs. A crack or break in a lumbar vertebra is usually responsible, resulting in two related conditions – spondylolysis and spondylolisthesis.

Microfracture

Compression forces cause the flat end plate of the vertebra, where it joins the disk, to crack. A small piece of an articular process may be broken off. This is typically caused by combined extension and rotation forces.

Compression fracture

Usually, the front of a vertebra collapses further than the back, so that the vertebra is wedge-shaped, making the spine appear humped.

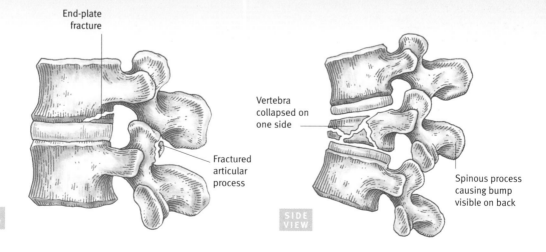

End-plate fracture

Fractured articular process

Vertebra collapsed on one side

Spinous process causing bump visible on back

SIDE VIEW

SIDE VIEW

Spondylolysis

This condition is a crack across the neural arch of a vertebra. In some instances, it is congenital, although the abnormality does not become apparent until the child is about six years old. Members of a family in which spondylosis is present are roughly 25 percent more likely to suffer from lower back pain than others. Spondylolysis can also result from an injury, usually after several falls onto the backside, or through overuse (*see p. 51*).

Spondylolisthesis

This condition is easier to identify because the neural arch separates. The vertebra shifts out of place, usually forward. Most cases develop from spondylolysis; the crack in the vertebra becomes a break as a result of excessive stresses and strains. Sometimes the vertebra slips gradually as the facet joints wear with age. This degenerative spondylolisthesis generally affects people aged 50 or over – it affects women more than men and African Americans more than Caucasians.

The displacement can be slight and without pain. If a shift is discovered in a growing child, X-ray monitoring every six months or so detects further movement. If the slip becomes severe, an abnormal shape due to shortening of the lower back may develop. The bones move most rapidly between the ages of 10 and 15. Once growth stops, the vertebrae are unlikely to slip further. Young people with spondylolisthesis should avoid contact sports and activities with a high risk of back injury.

Severe cases of both conditions may be treated with a fusion operation (*see p. 110*); decompression (*see p. 109*) in the older patient is usually enough. For milder cases, strengthening the postural stabilizing muscles will help.

Structural defects

Some back problems are caused by defects in the structure of the spine. A few are clearly apparent at birth, but many only become noticeable as a child grows. Some can be so mild that they come to light only on an X-ray when the patient's back is examined for an unrelated condition.

Functional scoliosis

This is a sideways curve of the spine, commonly caused by legs of unequal length, resulting in the pelvis tilting to one side. The spine compensates for the scoliosis by bending slightly toward the higher side to bring the level of the shoulders and the head back to horizontal.

Ten percent of the population have a difference in leg length of ⅖in (1cm) or more. Although this inequality causes a pelvic tilt and a mild compensatory curve of the spine, it rarely leads to problems, except perhaps in athletes who frequently put their spines under stress.

People with sciatica or an acute disk protrusion in the lower back, may try to minimize the disk pressure by bending sideways. Known as "sciatic scoliosis," this disappears when the protrusion resolves. Long-term sufferers may need exercises as well as manipulation to correct shortened muscles and stiff ligaments.

Structural scoliosis

True structural scoliosis (*see p. 54*) arises either in infancy, when it can be very severe, or during early adolescence. Vertebrae become narrower on one side so the spine leans towards that side and rotates. Spinal braces and supports worn during the growing phase can prevent excessive deformity. If your child's back seems crooked (look at the bare back as the child stands up straight and bends

Spondylolysis and spondylolisthesis

Initially, spondylolysis is just a minor crack across the narrow bridge of bone between the spinous and inferior articular processes and the transverse and superior articular processes. In spondylolisthesis, this crack widens to a break, allowing the vertebra to slip out of line. The illustrations below and right show the difference between the two conditions. When it slips, the vertebra may press against a nerve, causing pain along the path of the nerve.

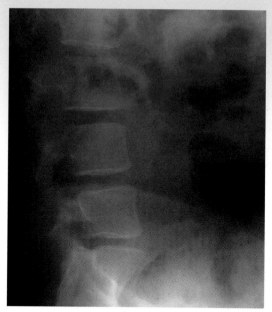

Spondylolisthesis
This X-ray above illustrates spondylolisthesis in the lumbar spine. Note how a vertebra has slipped out of line.

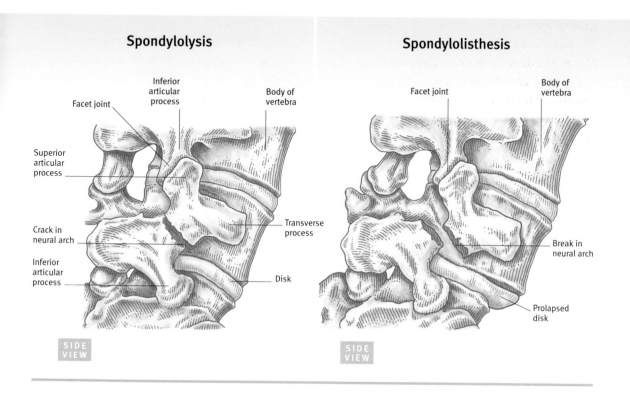

Spondylolysis

Facet joint

Inferior articular process

Body of vertebra

Superior articular process

Crack in neural arch

Inferior articular process

Transverse process

Disk

SIDE VIEW

Spondylolisthesis

Facet joint

Body of vertebra

Break in neural arch

Prolapsed disk

SIDE VIEW

Postural deformities

Abnormalities in the structure of the vertebrae can affect the spine and result in a deformed posture. For example, in scoliosis the vertebrae are narrow on one side, so the spine leans over to that side, and often twists back again a little higher up. In Scheuermann's disease, or adolescent osteochondritis, the vertebrae that are narrow at the front have the effect of making the spine hunch forward.

Scoliosis

The X-ray on the right shows a spine severely deformed by scoliosis. Milder scoliosis may be apparent only when the person bends forward, and a rib hump shows up prominently on one side.

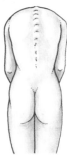 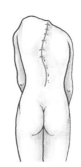

Normal spine   **Deformed spine**

BACK VIEW

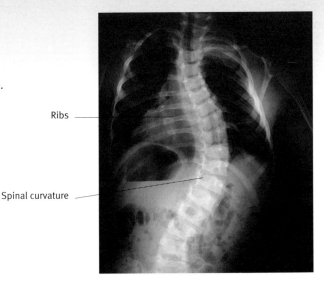

Ribs

Spinal curvature

Adolescent osteochondritis

The uneven, roughened edges of the vertebrae in the X-ray on the right can lead to wedging of the thoracic vertebrae. This makes the midback more hunched.

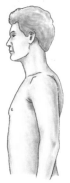 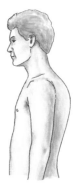

Normal spine   **Kyphotic spine**

SIDE VIEW

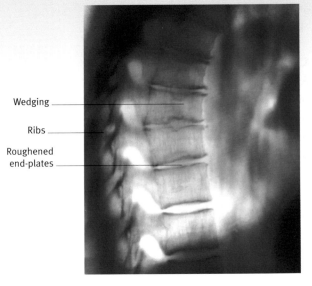

Wedging

Ribs

Roughened end-plates

forward), or one shoulder blade seems more prominent than the other, consult your doctor. Occasionally, the deformity may be severe enough to require surgery (*see p. 111*).

Mild scoliosis might produce no discomfort or pain initially. However, later in life, the unequal stresses and strains can accumulate and produce a general ache in any part of the back, shoulders, or neck. Also, chronic muscular tension patterns can set in. Joints between the vertebrae will degenerate earlier than usual. Most people, however, go through life with no greater incidence of backache than their counterparts with a straight spine.

Adolescent osteochondritis

This causes an excessively round-shouldered appearance or a humpback profile (*see left*). Also called Scheuermann's disease, it tends to occur in adolescents and frequently develops without any accompanying backache. The condition shows up on X-rays as mottled and roughened end plates in the midspine. There is no truly effective treatment other than corrective postural exercises. The abnormal curvature will stop when the skeleton stops growing. Rarely is it severe enough to require spinal bracing or surgery.

Congenital defects

A few children are born with defects. In spina bifida, the spinal cord is exposed or protected only by a thin membrane. It is always identified at birth or during pregnancy through prenatal screening. In the harmless spina bifida occulta, bone growth is absent from the neural arch.

Other defects occur in the lower back. For example, the lowest lumbar vertebra may fuse with the first sacral segment, so four lumbar segments can move instead of five. Such congenital defects rarely cause problems.

Postural pain

This is probably one of the most common causes of chronic backache. Postural pain may be caused by prolonged standing, sitting, or lying when one muscle or a group of muscles or ligaments are kept tense for a sustained period. The ligaments supporting the joints will start to hurt if you apply unequal, excessive, or sustained forces through the joints. See Chapter 8 for advice on posture.

Hollow back and swayback syndrome

Hollow back is a way of standing in which the abdomen is held forward, while the pelvis is tilted forward, so the lower back is arched. In swayback, the abdomen and pelvis slouch forward in front of the normal line of gravity (*see p. 140*).

They occur in some people with very flexible joints and others who let their abdominal muscles slacken with disuse so their pelvis tilts forward. Extra weight around the midriff adds to the strain. Pregnant women are particularly at risk.

They cause lower back pain, which may come from ligaments under tension in front of the lower back or from facet joint compression in the spine. The pain may radiate to the lower abdomen and hips. It may also reach the buttocks and upper thighs, particularly after standing for a long time.

The problem develops slowly and insidiously. You may never experience an acute episode of pain though you may feel sharp twinges, particularly when you change position. The simple cause of this back pain is often missed, but the cure usually lies in improved posture and simple exercises.

Kissing spines

This is a result of hollow back in which the tips of adjacent spinous processes touch each other and are compressed if the position is maintained for

Phases of disk degeneration

Disks are composed mostly of water, but they dry out with age. The gradual process of desiccation is hardly noticeable until around the age of 30, when the outer layers of the annulus fibrosus begins to degenerate and crack. The pulpy gel in the nucleus pulposus dries out gradually, which means that the disks of people around the age of 70 are much stiffer and less elastic. Although disk protrusions are less common by this age, thin disks can cause problems, particularly for the facet joints.

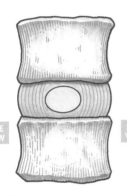

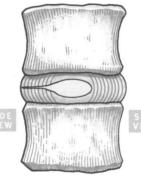

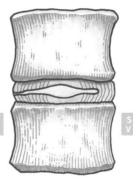

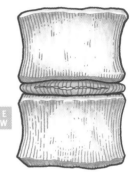

Stage 1
(20 to 30 years)
The nucleus pulposus of the disk is still healthy. During this period, hardly any fluid is lost from the pulpy gel.

Stage 2
(30 to 40 years)
The outer fibers are stiffer, with cracks developing in the annulus. The fluid content of the nucleus constantly decreases.

Stage 3
(40 to 50 years)
There is a progressive loss of fluid from the pulpy gel of the nucleus. The inner layers of the annulus have collapsed.

Stage 4
(50 to 70 years)
The disk becomes both thinner and drier, with a very much smaller nucleus. The annulus is stiff and inelastic.

any prolonged period of time. This compression tends to cause a more sharply localized pain. Improved posture will help, but injections or even surgery may be needed.

Forward head position

People who lean over a desk for long periods with their head bent forward put continuous strain on their upper back and neck muscles. This can be aggravated by hunching, which puts a chronic strain on the trapezius muscles in the shoulders.

This posture would normally strain the muscles rather than the ligaments. It leads to aching in the neck, shoulder, and shoulder blade area which develops after some hours and can be relieved by getting up and moving around. However, the time comes when this no longer relieves the pain and a pattern of chronic muscular tension sets in. Neck strain may occasionally lead to tension headaches, which develop late in the day or in the evening.

The aging spine

As the spine ages, the bones and disks degenerate. Bones usually lose calcium and grow bony spurs. The disks gradually grow drier and thinner (*see above*), and the ligaments may weaken or stiffen. The degeneration, which is also called spondylosis or osteoarthritis, is visible in X-rays in about 75 percent of the population over 50 years old.

It usually affects the lower neck and the lower lumbar spine first. Although rarely a direct cause of backache, aging can lead to conditons such as lateral canal stenosis, osteoporosis, Paget's disease and facet syndrome.

Lateral canal stenosis

Vertebrae grow bony spurs, or osteophytes, which may make the central or lateral spinal canal much narrower. Known as stenosis, this can result in pinched nerves (*see below and Spinal stenosis, p. 59*).

Lateral canal stenosis

Bony spurs, or osteophytes, form a protruding rim around the edge of the vertebra and the facet joints. They may encroach on the lateral canal (foramen) causing stenosis (constriction), and can result in a pinched nerve.

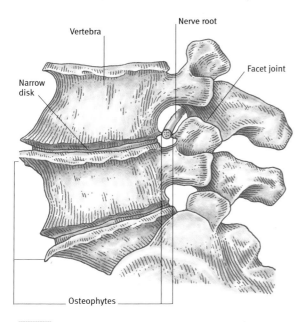

Nerve root

Vertebra

Facet joint

Narrow disk

Osteophytes

SIDE VIEW

Lateral canal stenosis may cause pain in the arm or leg, depending on where the nerve is pinched. The pain may not be constant – you may feel it as you bend back or twist your spine, when the canal is narrower. You will experience intermittent pain down the leg, perhaps with pins and needles or numbness. A protruding disk, which causes a more constant pain, further narrows the lateral spinal canal, or foramen.

Improved stability may help the condition, so seek advice on posture and exercises to tighten your muscles. Severe cases of lateral canal stenosis may need decompression surgery (*see p. 109*).

Osteoporosis

Bones gradually become thin as they lose their calcium and mineral structure but the process occurs almost invariably with aging and tends to accelerate with disuse and immobility. The demineralization tends to speed up after menopause or after long-term use of oral steroids.

Prevention is best: remain as active as possible in your later years and, starting as a young adult, get enough calcium and vitamin D, either in your food or as supplements. If you are developing compression fractures of the spine (*see p. 58*) then bisphosphonates can restore bone mineral.

A family history of osteoporosis, late onset of puberty, early menopause, smoking, anorexia nervosa, and malabsorption are all risk factors that make it advisable to get your bone density checked with a DEXA scan. Hormone replacement therapy (HRT) is often recommended for postmenopausal women if there are no contraindications.

Paget's disease

This rare disease tends to occur in the elderly and results in irregular resorption and remodeling of bone and greater bone density. The first symptoms may be a pain in the hip, thigh, or arm, since the disease tends to affect the whole skeleton, not just the vertebrae. An X-ray should show the irregular increases in bone density (*see below*).

FACET SYNDROME

One consequence of having thinner disks is that the facet joints are jammed closer together and so are put under much greater pressure than normal. The joints can then become irritated and inflamed, causing the joint capsule (*see p. 12*) to swell and to press on a nerve root.

In the lower back

In its early stages, facet joint disease can cause pain in the lower spine when you stand for long periods and sharp twinges as you change position. Some positions, such as lying on your front, may be hard to adopt. As facet syndrome advances, you may suffer from a continuous backache with acute phases. Symptoms may be worse in cold weather.

Improved posture, exercises, physical therapy, or acupuncture can help the early stages, but facet joint injections (*see p. 105*) may be needed to relieve inflammation. Manipulation may help with

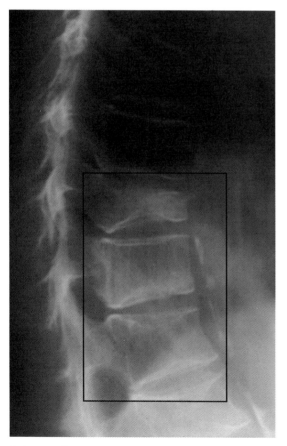

Osteoporosis
The wedge shape of the crushed vertebra is typical of a compression fracture caused by osteoporosis.

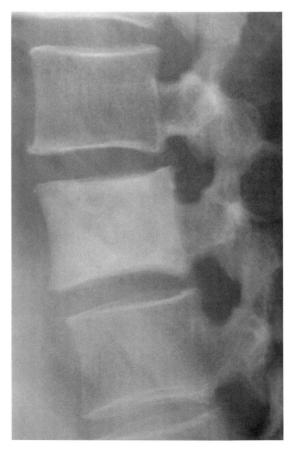

Paget's disease
This X-ray shows the irregular thickening of the body of the vertebra in Paget's disease.

acute episodes but radiofrequency denervation (*see p. 105*) is the best treatment in the long term. Surgery, such as lateral decompression (*see p. 109*) may help a trapped nerve root.

In the neck

Similar problems can occur in the neck region. As well as the aching accompanied by sharp twinges, you also might experience numbness or pins and needles in your hands if osteoarthritic change is narrowing the foramen.

Other complications may include disturbed balance, ringing in the ears, headaches, and pain referred to the face, side of the neck, and ear. If you are over 60, the vertebral artery can be affected, causing dizzy spells and even blackouts when you move your neck or arm in certain ways.

In the elderly, the neck seems to be exempt from the stabilization that benefits the rest of the spine. Careful posture, massage, exercises, and acupuncture (*see p. 158*), may provide some relief from facet syndrome, but are unlikely cure it. Radiofrequency facet denervation (*see p. 105*) is, however, very effective. Surgery to the cervical spine is risky and is therefore only undertaken if the spinal cord is threatened or with progressive weakness.

Spinal stenosis

The central spinal canal can sometimes become too narrow, reducing the flow of blood to the nerves supplying both legs or one side only. This stenosis is not so common in the neck since the canal is wider at the top.

Degenerative change

In middle-aged or elderly people, osteophytes (bony spurs) may grow, narrowing the spinal canal and affecting the nerves. You feel pins and needles, numbness, and heaviness or pain in both legs when you walk or run. Sitting, bending forward, or crouching widen the spinal canal and bring relief. Bending backward or twisting narrows the canal further and causes sharp pain. You may need to undergo a decompression operation (*see p. 109*).

Congenital traits

People born with a spinal canal that is narrower than normal are more at risk of nerve compression and of developing chronic back problems or sciatica if a disk ruptures or herniates. Problems can afflict young adults but more often affect the middle-aged and elderly. In very severe cases, decompression surgery may be needed (*see p. 105*).

Inflammation and disease

A very small percentage of back problems are the result of inflammatory conditions, such as ankylosing spondylitis or rheumatoid arthritis, or by a cancer that either invades the spine or develops within it. Very rarely, problems may be caused by arachnoiditis (adhesions inside the dural sleeve around the nerve root) or by infections, such as brucellosis or tuberculosis.

Ankylosing spondylitis

This condition tends to occur in young adults – affecting men more severely than women. Joints become inflamed and ligaments calcify to stiffen the spine (*see p. 61*). Little is known about its cause but the disease usually affects the sacroiliac joint first, and advances gradually over several years. Eventually, the inflammation affects the joints between the ribs and the midspine, which reduces chest expansion and makes breathing difficult.

The first symptoms of ankylosing spondylitis are pain and stiffness in the lower back and are

Causes of central canal stenosis

The spinal canal varies in size and shape along its entire length: it is widest in the neck, before many nerves have branched out. Even a small reduction in diameter of the spinal canal can result in severe pain and other symptoms as blood supply to the nerves is reduced. It may be narrowed by a protruding disk or by osteophytes. Some people are born with canals that are narrow, triangular or cloverleaf-shaped. These do not leave enough room for the spinal nerves and can cause severe pain in later life.

Normal spinal canal

The canal is normally open and unobstructed, allowing enough space for the spinal cord.

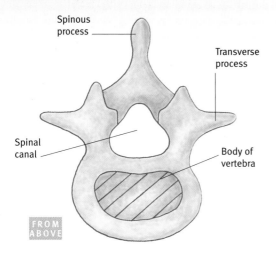

Disk protrusion

When a disk protrudes, it encroaches on the central spinal canal and presses on the spinal nerves.

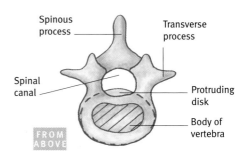

Osteophytes

Bony spurs called osteophytes grow on the vertebrae and into the canal, causing it to become narrow.

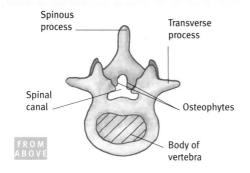

Congenitally narrow canal

The growth of the vertebrae before birth determines the diameter of the canal.

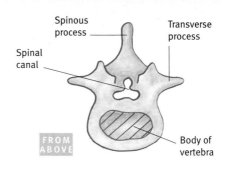

generally worst upon waking. You may find it difficult to bend forward and your hip joints will be stiff. The pain is usually relieved by moderate exercise (*see Chapter 7*).

It is important to identify this condition as early as possible to prevent deterioration in your posture and mobility. Your doctor will prescribe some anti-inflammatory drugs and refer you to a physical therapist for specific exercises to maintain your mobility.

Rheumatoid arthritis

This inflammatory condition usually starts in the small joints of the hands and feet and progresses until it affects the larger joints, such as the knees, hips, elbows, and shoulders. Rheumatoid arthritis does not usually attack the spine until later in its course, and then it usually affects the neck. By the time it reaches the spine, the diagnosis should have been made.

It is unlikely that your doctor could mistake rheumatoid arthritis for any other spinal disorder, because it will be affecting many other joints before it reaches the spine. If your doctor mentions arthritis when discussing your back, however, he is probably referring to the normal signs of wear and tear associated with aging (*see pp. 56–59*).

Infection

This is a rare cause of backache these days. The pain and aching usually develop insidiously over a period of weeks and months and are not relieved by either lying down or resting. If a large abscess develops in or around the bone or disk, the area is often extremely tender and local muscle might go into spasm at the slightest touch. By the time the infection reaches this severity, there would be other signs of illness, such as a fever or general malaise.

Occasionally, there may be an infection in the disk itself, called "diskitis." Some people may suffer from a temporary "diskitis," after the use of chymopapain (*see p. 107*). This produces a deep, severe backache, which is exquisitely painful with any movement. The treatment for an infection in or around the spine is a specific antibiotic taken intravenously, injected directly into the muscles over several weeks, or it may be by mouth.

Ankylosing spondylitis

This disease causes the disks and ligaments of the spine to harden gradually and become like bone, making the spine stiff and inflexible. This extreme stiffness results in a person hunching forward with a flat chest and a rounded spine.

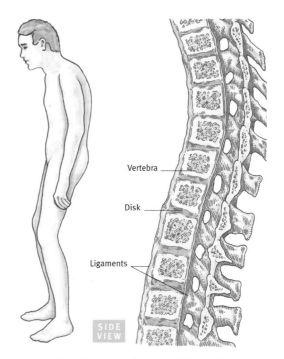

Vertebra

Disk

Ligaments

SIDE VIEW

Posture resulting from ankylosing spondylitis

Close-up of affected spine

4

Getting Help

Time and a change of routine are the essential healers for recovery from an acute attack of back pain. Rest, relax, take some form of pain relief if you need to, and adjust your day-to-day living. As soon as the worst pain has passed, try doing some gentle exercise or have a massage but it helps to know you are dealing with a simple physical strain first.

A proper assessment is necessary before reassurance and explanation can be given. The person in the best position to start the process is your doctor: she has access to all your medical records and

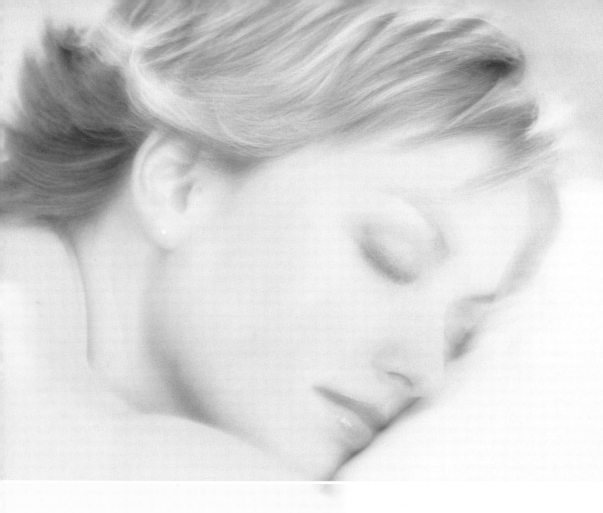

can refer you to the appropriate specialist or therapist if needed.
Consult your doctor – particularly if you are worried or if this is your
first attack of back pain. If you are prone to recurrent back pain, you
will probably know what your doctor would advise, so you may not
gain very much from seeing him each time. If you have been through
this stage and it proved unsatisfactory, try a recommended physical
therapist, although you may need to approach specialists through
your doctor, and it is wise to keep your doctor informed.

Who should I consult?

You should see your doctor (*see p. 74*) if this is your first ever attack of back pain and it is not easing, or if you are in severe pain, or if you are an urgent case (*see below*). You should also see your doctor if you cannot match your condition with the types of acute episode in Chapter 3.

If you wish to consult a practitioner other than your doctor, I would advise the following courses of action, depending on the type and severity of the pain you are experiencing:

• Consult an osteopath, chiropractor, musculoskeletal physician, or manipulative physical therapist if your pain is bearable but is not easing after 10 to 14 days, or if you are in a hurry to get better.

• If you are prone to back or neck pain that is frequent and recurring, see a physical therapist who has received training in postural stabilization for prevention of back pain and general care of the back, or consult a musculoskeletal physician.

• If you have chronic back or neck pain, consult a specialist in musculoskeletal, orthopedic, or rheumatological medicine. Alternatively, visit a pain clinic or try one of the various ways of coping with chronic pain (*see Chapter 9*).

See a doctor urgently

Seek medical attention as soon as possible in the the following instances of back pain:

• Unrelenting pain. This back pain is not made particularly better or worse by any one movement or position. It also increases steadily over weeks and months, troubling you both day and night.

• Deteriorating muscles. A profound weakness or wasting away of some of the muscles in either one or both legs or arms (as opposed to a temporary inability to move because of the pain) implies considerable nerve damage. It may be accompanied by a weak bladder, incontinence or loss of the sensation to urinate, or sudden loss of sexual function. The bowel may also be affected.

• General ailing health. Your back pain has become a painful highlight against a background of feeling unwell for some weeks or months – you have been increasingly tired, losing your appetite, mildly feverish at times, or losing weight.

• Loss of sensation. Widespread numbness and pins and needles in the legs, arms, or crotch area may indicate a serious problem such as a large disk prolapse affecting spinal nerves. The numbness must be distinguished from the temporary pins and needles caused by sitting or lying awkwardly.

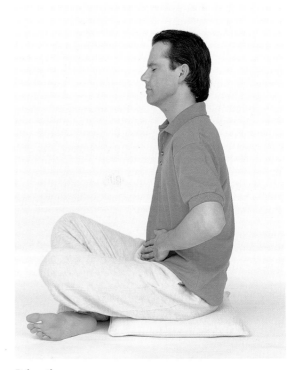

Relaxation
Sit still, with your back straight and your legs crossed, and relax your mind and body. Place your hand on your diaphragm to help you focus on your breathing.

Don't panic

If you have an acute attack of pain, try to get your problem into perspective. Ask yourself:
• Is the pain so severe that you need a prescription for strong pain medication?
• Is it bearable if you find a comfortable position and relax into it?
• After a while in a comfortable position, is it less painful when you move again?
• Are you content to wait for a natural recovery? See pp. 66–74 for useful tips for reducing the pain and improving your ability to move freely.

Stay calm and in control

After almost any physical shock to the body, rest is a natural part of first aid. In an acute attack of back pain, rest may be necessary initially. Resting for too long, however, slows recovery and could prevent a full recovery, since the affected part may stiffen up and muscles may weaken. If the pain does not immobilize you, reduce some activities such as carrying heavy objects, heavy manual work, and prolonged driving or sitting, until the pain eases.

Relax and breathe easily

Try to relax mentally and physically (*see Simple relaxation, p. 68*). The key to relaxing your muscles is correct breathing. We are rarely conscious of how we breathe and so a fixed habit of shallow breathing, tense diaphragm, and a tight jaw and throat can develop.

When you breathe in, let your mouth stay open in a relaxed way; instead of simply expanding your chest, breathe deeply so your diaphragm descends and your abdomen rises. Your chest hardly needs to rise at all – it is the diaphragm that should provide the automatic rhythm. Do not try to

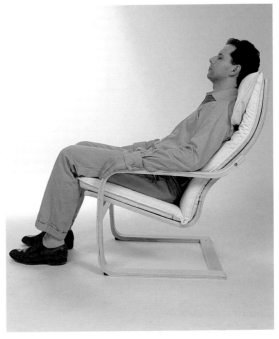

A rocking chair
Sitting in a rocking chair can help you get away from the stresses and strains of everyday life. The gentle and calming movement is soothing when you are in pain and can help to relieve a backache.

breathe in too deeply or too quickly. Concentrate on exhalation. Let your jaw relax, your mouth fall open, and your chest sink when you breathe out. It often helps to let go with a prolonged and audible sigh. Imagine the muscles in each part of your body letting go of the tension. Start with the face, then the neck and work downward. Repeat the process, checking every area.

Keep your spine straight

Lying flat on your back reduces the pressure on your spine to a minimum. However, it may not be the most comfortable position. The important point is for the spine to be straight. There are various advantages to this: you take the strain off the joints and disks, which will relieve pain and may help the condition ease up. When you sit or bend, the painful area must still bear its normal load of body weight.

Pain can often make muscles seize up in a protective spasm (if you can't move, you can't be hurt). You can reduce the spasm by lying down. Lying on your front, face down, may be as good, if not better, as lying on your side. However, its effects vary from person to person. If a disk is protruding toward the back of the spine, this position may be too painful initially. The same is true if you have an inflamed or sprained facet joint. In both cases, try the Fowler position (*see below*). This position gently stretches the lower back, opening the facet joints slightly and accommodating the protruding disk rather than pinching it. Consequently, the protective muscle tension is encouraged to relax. Gradually lower your legs by using fewer pillows, once the acute spasm has passed.

Sitting

A sitting position may be the most comfortable but it can slow recovery because the pressure on the disks will be 150 percent (*see p. 143*). When sitting up, keep your back straight if your pain is caused by a protruding disk. You may slouch as you sit so that the disk is no longer pressing on a nerve, but the weight of your spine will still press down on the disk, slowing its natural resolution.

Resting your spine

Try these positions to find the best one for you. If you prefer lying on your side, one side may be more comfortable than the other.

Lie on a firm bed base and a firm, but not too hard, mattress (*see p. 147*). When lying on your back, do not use a pillow unless you are uncomfortable without one; even then you should use only one pillow, otherwise your spine may flex too much. Special pillows for helping neck pain are available (*see p. 147*). Try also a pillow under your knees. An adjustable bed allows you to elevate the lower section and adopt the Fowler position.

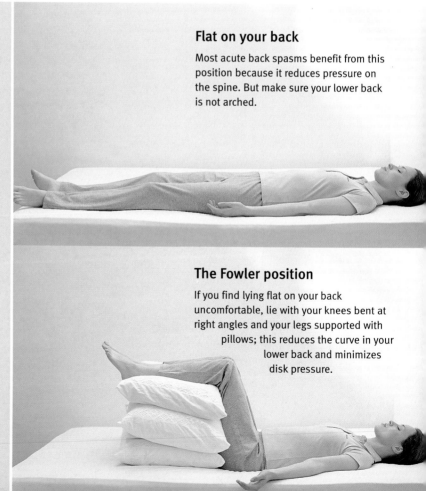

Flat on your back

Most acute back spasms benefit from this position because it reduces pressure on the spine. But make sure your lower back is not arched.

The Fowler position

If you find lying flat on your back uncomfortable, lie with your knees bent at right angles and your legs supported with pillows; this reduces the curve in your lower back and minimizes disk pressure.

Neck pain

Acute neck pain may hurt when you hold your head up, so spend the first day or two lying flat to avoid added stress. When sleeping, tuck a twisted pillow or a rolled and twisted towel around your neck as if it were a thick scarf (*see below*).

To rest or not to rest

There is no virtue in prolonged bed rest: you shouldn't stay in bed for more than two to three days. Recent evidence shows that moving as early as your pain allows leads to a better short and long-term outcome. If you need a few days' rest, do not get up and help around the house. This will undo all the beneficial effects of rest. Enjoy being cared

for if you have the help. To relieve any boredom you may feel, listen to music, read books, watch television, or call friends and family. Eat your meals lying on your side or propped up on one elbow. Do not be tempted to sit up. Avoid straining on the toilet. Get up as soon as you can and do not be afraid to get moving again.

Relaxation and pain relief

Severe pain causes your muscles to go into spasm, which in turn increases your pain. Relief from pain not only makes you more comfortable, it enables you to get moving again. Try remedies such as heat or ice, massage, medicines, hand-held massagers,

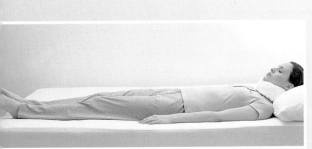

Supporting your neck

Roll up a small towel into a sausage shape, then place it around your neck. This acts as a soft collar and prevents your head from lolling to either side at night.

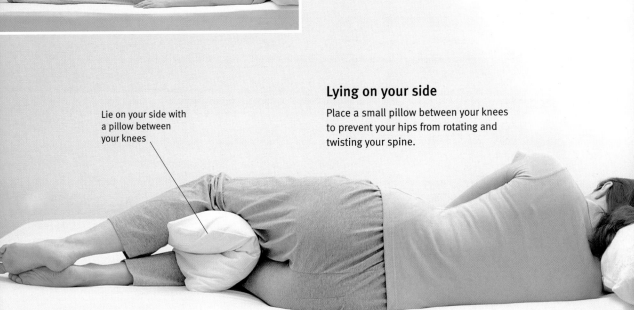

Lie on your side with a pillow between your knees

Lying on your side

Place a small pillow between your knees to prevent your hips from rotating and twisting your spine.

Simple relaxation

Muscle tension may be a response to a worrying or irritating situation, or to pain or postural stress. Whatever the reason, it can be a major cause of back and neck pain, and one that you can often avoid if you teach yourself to recognize the danger signs and relax before it is too late.

Some muscle tension is, of course, essential for every move you make, but if you practice relaxation you will soon become aware of unnecessary tension in your body and learn how to release it. Before long you will notice yourself hunched over the steering wheel while driving, or gripping the receiver too tight when on the phone. You will notice that you are sitting in a tense position during a meeting, or while feeding a baby. Whatever the demands on your life, you can learn to reduce the stress factor.

The simple exercises described below make use of the principle that if you tighten one group of muscles the opposite group will relax. Set aside a little time for them each day and you will learn to release tension busy for other, more strenuous exercises.

How to relax

Remove your shoes and loosen tight clothing. Listen to soothing music if it helps reduce tension. Lie on your back on the floor or a firm bed with one pillow under your head, your arms by your sides or resting on your stomach, and your legs uncrossed.

If your back aches or feels very tense, put a pillow under your knees. If your back is acutely painful or if you are heavily pregnant, you will probably find it more comfortable to lie on your side with your lower arm behind you, your upper knee bent forward on a pillow, and your lower leg straight.

If you do not want to lie down, relax in an armchair. Keep your head and arms fully supported and your legs uncrossed.

1 Start by pulling your shoulders down toward your feet. Lengthen the gap between your ears and your shoulders. Stop and feel the new position – it should be easy and comfortable.

2 Push your elbows out. Stop when your arms are comfortable and register this position.

3 Lengthen your fingers – stretch them to the fingertips and stretch your thumbs. Stop, and let them rest outstretched.

4 Tighten your buttocks and rotate your legs so that your feet roll out. Let your legs feel heavy.

5 Move your knees around if you want to. Stop. Let your legs feel heavy again.

6 Push your feet gently down away from you. Stop and just let your feet hang comfortably from your ankles.

7 Press your body into the support behind you, if you are in a chair. Stop, then just let it sink into the support and enjoy this feeling.

8 Press your head back into the pillow or the back of the chair. Stop. Let the whole weight of your head sink into the pillow.

9 Close your eyes gently. Let your eyelids feel heavy. Open your mouth so that you unclench your teeth. Close it gently. Push your tongue down on the bottom teeth, then let it rest in the middle of your mouth. Let your forehead feel smooth and comfortable, with no worry lines.

10 Be aware of your breathing. It will probably be slower now that you are relaxed. Be aware of taking air to the base of your lungs as you breathe in and then sigh your breath out slowly. Continue breathing easily and comfortably while you rest for 10 to 15 minutes, or for as long as you can.

and rubs. When your pain is temporarily relieved, start to resume your normal activities – do not be afraid of the pain since you will not be harming anything or causing more damage.

Heat or ice

Place a hot-water bottle or microwavable "wheat" pack against the most painful part of your back. Its soothing effect may relax tight muscles and relieve pain. In general, avoid hot baths because you may be struck with severe pain when try to get out.

Ice is good for relieving pain and reducing muscle tension. Use either a package of frozen peas wrapped in a thin cloth, or several ice cubes crushed in a pack. Apply the ice over the painful area for 15 minutes, and repeat every two to three hours.

Massage

Having a massage can help relax the muscles as well as relieve pain, and the tension brought on by a person's fears and his or her voluntary reaction to pain. A willing partner or friend doesn't have to be an expert to give a soothing but firm massage, just sensitive hands. A calm, reassuring attitude to touching a friend or partner is comforting. For advice on giving a massage, see pages 70–71. Alternatively, you can relieve your own pain with acupressure (*see p. 72*).

Medicines

Of the common pain remedies, such as aspirin, ibuprofen, or acetaminophen, I tend to favor aspirin. There is a risk of gastric irritation if it is taken for a prolonged period. You should definitely avoid it if you have had a peptic ulcer or indigestion.

If you take the full prescribed dosage of aspirin regularly it will not only reduce your pain but will also reduce inflammation. This latter effect is very important in conditions involving inflammation, such as facet joint irritation or swelling around the dural root sleeve.

Aspirin or ibuprofen or other NSAIDs (non-steroidal antinflammatories) may also counter the irritant effect of a protruding disk and can reduce the inflammation caused by local internal bleeding in cases where the muscles, ligaments, or joints have been damaged.

Lying on your side

If you are most comfortable lying on your side, make sure you support your head to take the pressure off your neck.

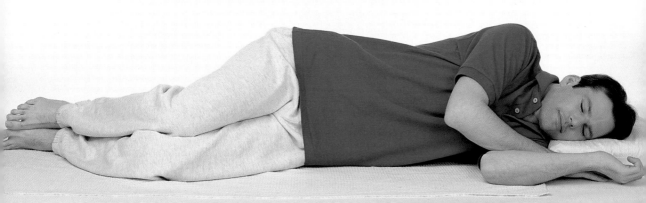

Relaxation through massage

Massage is an excellent way of relaxing tired and aching muscles and anyone can do it: contrary to popular belief, you do not need professional training. In some parts of the world, children learn to give and accept massage as part of their general upbringing. We may have lost this tradition in the West and opted for more modern forms of healing, but most people would prefer a massage to a course of tranquilizers. Massage is also an ideal way of relieving a backache during labor.

The general effect of a massage is to relax the muscles and to stimulate the circulation. The overall mental effect can be both relaxing and stimulating. A massage does not have to be extremely painful, but nor should it be absolutely painless.

Particularly tense areas around the neck and shoulders may be trigger points, which are often painful when pressed firmly (*see p. 48*). The tender areas should be massaged until they feel relaxed. If the muscle tightens or goes into spasm in response to pressure, then either the massage is too hard, or you are not able to tolerate that level of pain. Massage will help you to identify areas of tension and this knowledge, as well as the massage itself, may help you relax.

Giving a massage

Choose a well-heated room and a comfortable yet firm surface to lie on. Most beds are too soft for a massage, so it is generally better to lay a blanket or towel on the floor and ask your partner to lie down on his front.

Make sure that your hands are warm, and rub a little oil into your palms. Make and break contact gently, and massage with firm, rhythmic strokes, concentrating particularly on the tense areas.

Massaging the back

These instructions are for a complete back massage. If the person you are massaging suffers from aching muscles in just one region of the back, concentrate on that area. Unless otherwise specified, always work from the top of the spine downward. Start with strokes from the shoulders and work down to the midback or start at the midback and work down to the buttocks.

1 Start with a few long, gentle strokes down the center of the back from the base of the neck to the buttocks, and lightly up the sides.

2 Knead the shoulder muscles, gradually increasing the pressure. Work up the neck to the base of the skull.

3 Massage the shoulder blade area and the muscles around the mid spine. Use small circular movements, mixed with longer, gentle strokes.

4 Apply thumb pressure down the bands of muscle beside the spine, starting at the neck. When you reach the midback, glide your hands up to the neck again and repeat. Follow with finger pressure on the same bands of muscle.

5 Apply hand pressure across the shoulders and right down the back to the buttocks.

6 Knead the large muscles of the lower back and buttocks.

7 Apply thumb pressure down the bands of muscle next to the spine, from the midback to the buttocks.

8 Work with circling movements on either side of the spine.

9 Apply pressure with your hand, starting at the midback. Then, using the index and middle fingers of each hand, press firmly on the bands of muscles beside the spine in short, overlapping strokes. Apply firm strokes down the back with your hands flat, and bring the massage to a finish with long, soothing strokes.

Basic techniques

Various strokes are involved in giving a massage. These are either appropriate to different stages of the massage or to different areas of the body. The techniques shown here are some of the most useful for massaging the back; your partner will be able to tell you which are the most relaxing.

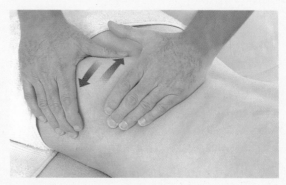

Kneading
Squeeze the flesh gently between your fingers and thumbs in rippling movements, or between the heel of your hand and your fingers, as if kneading dough.

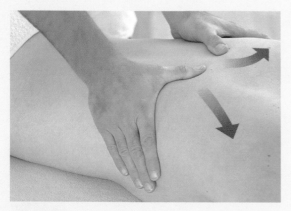

Long strokes
Start a massage with gentle, sweeping strokes covering a wide area. They spread the oil and prepare your partner for long, firmer strokes. Use your whole hand flat on the skin and make large circular movements. Start the massage with very little pressure and gradually increase it.

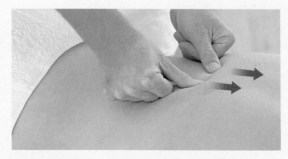

Thumb pressure
This massage is good for bands of tense muscle. Press firmly with your thumb in a long, smooth stroke.

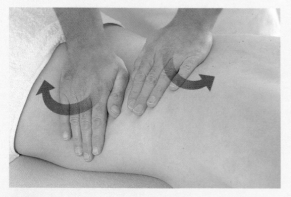

Circling
Press firmly, making circular movements. Try to build up a rhythm, without losing contact. On wider or more fleshy areas, use the heel of a hand and work in larger circles.

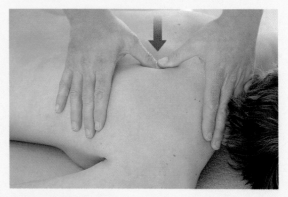

Hand or finger pressure
Place one thumb on the small tense nodules and the other on top. Press firmly and hold for 30 seconds. Repeat at other tender sites. You can use fingers instead of thumbs.

Acupressure

This is a method of massage that works on the same principle of stimulating influential points and meridians as acupuncture (*see p. 159*). The difference is that these points are stimulated by pressure – often with the thumb or finger – rather than with acupuncture needles. As a result you can safely try this yourself without having to go to a specialist.

There are three main points on the body for the relief of back pain and sciatica. Place the tip of one finger on one of the points indicated below. Press down hard and vibrate the finger rapidly but slightly for several minutes, or until the pain decreases. The subsequent relief from pain may last for only a few minutes, but sometimes it can last for several days.

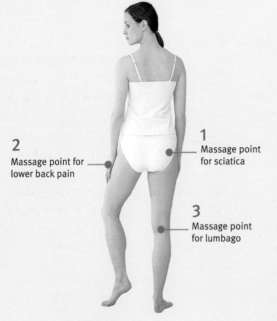

2
Massage point for lower back pain

1
Massage point for sciatica

3
Massage point for lumbago

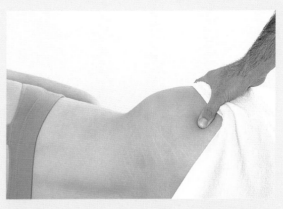

1 Sciatica
Lie down on your painless side with the affected leg half bent. Ask your partner to place a forefinger over the bony protrusion of the pelvis while keeping the thumb at right angles to the rest of the hand. The tip of the thumb will lie directly over the acupressure point.

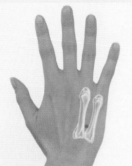

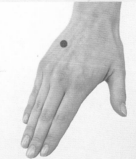

2 Lower back pain
Pain in the mid to lower back may be relieved by pressure on this point. From the knuckles of the ring finger and little finger on your right hand, slide your left forefinger toward the wrist until you feel a slight dip. The acupressure point lies about two thirds of the way down from the knuckles to the wrist.

3 Acute lumbago
To relieve intense lower back pain which is restricting movement, press in the middle of the fold behind your knee on either leg.

If over-the-counter remedies are not strong enough, ask your doctor for something stronger. Take the pills regularly, not sporadically, since the pain control is greater when blood levels are maintained.

Rubs

There are two basic types. Those with an active medicinal base, such as aspirin, are absorbed through the skin into the deeper layers of muscles. Those with strongly aromatic or irritant oils, such as mentholatum, create a burning sensation on the skin, which "distracts" the brain temporarily. The muscle relaxes once it is free of pain.

Most of the benefit probably comes from the fact that the oils are massaged into the skin. They may give some relief in mild to moderate pain but they neither last long enough nor are effective in alleviating the more severe attacks of pain.

Use your mind power

Practice the following sequence of four steps for 10 to 15 minutes three times a day. You will discover that you can help yourself regain a sense of control by becoming increasingly aware of your reactions to your back pain:

- Ask yourself – are you resentful and frustrated at this sudden and imposed limitation? If so, then ACCEPT where you are now. Give in to the pain. If you face it rather than run away, you will find it is not nearly so frightening.
- Are you bracing against the pain? The more you tense up, the worse you are making it – so RELAX.
- Are you thinking negatively? Are you saying to yourself "My back is broken" or "I'm going to be paralyzed" or "I'll never be able to get back to work or take that vacation"? If you think like this, you will certainly feel worse. So CONTROL your runaway thoughts immediately.
- Change your FOCUS. Direct your attention to a part of your body that does feel comfortable, such as your breathing rhythm or those warm muscles. Allow that sense of comfort to spread through your body. Now imagine yourself in your favorite place where you feel calm, happy, and secure – by the lake, on the beach, in a sunny meadow.

Day-to-day living

During an acute attack, you will have to adapt to a limited range of movements. While the pain is severe, move around as much as possible but follow the rules of back and neck care (*see Chapter 8*). Always think how you do something to reduce the buildup of pain or fatigue.

Start moving as soon as the pain begins to die down. After the initial severe pain has subsided (which varies from 12 to 24 hours to two or three days), start mobilizing exercises (*see p. 120*). These prevent your back from stiffening up. Some specifically help to ease the nucleus of the disk back toward the center; others gently open the facet joints.

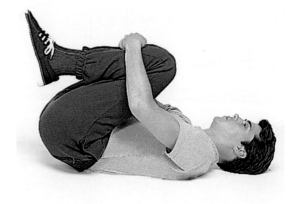

Relieve the pain
Some types of back pain can be eased if you lie on your back and gently hold your bent knees to your chest.

Returning to active daily life

You probably belong to the majority of people with acute back or neck pain who recover spontaneously within one month or thereabouts. Consequently, the chances are that, after a few days, you will want to get moving and return to your everyday life.

At this stage, it is important to follow the basic principles of back care (*see Chapter 8*). The tissues are still in the healing phase and will respond positively to normal movement. At times, you may feel stiffness, perhaps even marked discomfort, but remember that "hurt does not necessarily mean harm" as you get your joints and muscles working normally again.

Consulting your doctor

If this is your first bout of back pain, consult your doctor. Usually back pain is not an emergency, but do not expect an instant cure or instant relief. Your doctor will probably ask the following questions. Try to answer as fully and clearly as possible to help him make an accurate diagnosis.

- What were you doing when the pain started?
- Did the pain come on suddenly or did it build up gradually?
- Where do you feel it and where does it radiate?
- Is the pain sharp, dull, heavy, burning?
- What positions or movements relieve it, and which aggravate it?

Moving: respect the pain but do not fear it

By avoiding bending or sitting down for the first two hours of the day, sufferers of chronic back pain can significantly reduce their symptoms.

The advice given here may prevent painful twinges in the joints in your lower back. With practice, the movements can become fluent. Continue moving in this way, even when your back is not painful.

While your back is painful, avoid wearing clothes that are difficult to put on or take off, such as tight jeans. Use slip-on shoes rather than lace-ups.

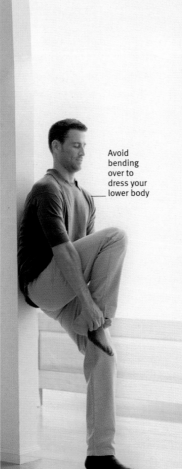

Avoid bending over to dress your lower body

Getting dressed

Avoid sitting down and bending over to put your clothes on, since this strains your back. Roll your clothes up so that you can put your arms or legs through quickly and easily. Stand on one leg (lean against a wall if necessary) and raise your knee to dress your lower half (*see left*).

Getting dressed lying down

Pull your knees up to your chest to get the clothes over your feet, then straighten your legs as you pull the clothes up.

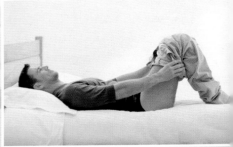

- Is the pain constant?
- Do you feel any numbness or pins and needles?
- Have you had similar episodes before?
- What kind of job do you do?
- What daily actions involve your back?

Describing your pain

If you can describe your pain, and its intensity, the doctor can make a more accurate diagnosis. Many adjectives can express the quality and severity of pain. Some describe the physical sensation: sharp, pulsating, shooting, stabbing. Perhaps your pain is gnawing, pulling, burning, searing, or stinging. Adjectives that reflect the feeling associated with pain may be more descriptive: tiring, wretched, sickening, miserable, frightful. Others can express the overall intensity of the pain you feel: dreadful, vicious, unbearable, terrible, or torturous.

Different types of pain have different causes, according to the tissues involved. A general, dull ache is often due to tense muscles or an irritation from deep within the spinal joints. A sharp and shooting pain may be caused by a pinched nerve and, as with lumbar and cervical radiculopathy, it may not be felt at the site of injury. A sharp but clearly defined pain which does not spread to any other sites comes from pinched tissues such as the skin or the lining on a bone.

A diffuse, burning sensation is often caused by a disturbance of the sympathetic nervous system,

Getting out of bed

Bring your knees up to about hip level and roll over on to your side. Lower your feet to the floor and use your arms to push yourself up into a sitting position. Reverse this procedure to get back into bed.

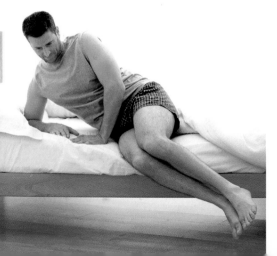

Getting in and out of an armchair

To sit down in a chair, stand with your back to the chair and your feet shoulder width apart, close to the edge of the chair. Keep your back straight and lower yourself slowly. Place your hands on the arms of the chair as soon as you can.

To get out of a chair, bring your feet as close as you can to the edge of the chair, if possible under the edge. At the same time, bring your buttocks vertically above your feet. Keep your knees shoulder width apart for good balance. Keep your spine straight, and place your hands on the arms of the chair. Slowly straighten your legs and push yourself out of the chair with your arms (*right*).

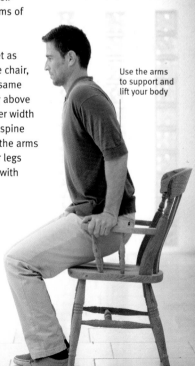

Use the arms to support and lift your body

which controls the involuntary and subconscious functions such as circulation and sweating. These nerves do not control any of your voluntary actions, so you would not notice any weakness accompanying the pain.

Preliminary treatment

After examining you (*see below*), the doctor will make a preliminary diagnosis. Since 94 percent of back pain is simply mechanical, five percent is nerve root pain, and one percent is possibly serious and requiring investigation, it likely that the doctor can explain the problem and provide reassurance. He may encourage a short period of rest with simple pain medication or muscle relaxants followed by mobilization (gradually increasing activity). The basic message will be: modify your activities, stay active, and do not fear the pain. As you get moving again, remember "hurt does not usually mean harm." Finally, you will be encouraged to return to work as soon as you can.

If you are in severe pain, you will probably need a strong analgesic to take regularly. Do not be afraid to ask for stronger pain medication and, if you have any worries about addiction, discuss them with your doctor. If you experience recurrent episodes of back pain, and your job entails lifting or carrying heavy objects, ask your doctor to communicate with your employer about a phased return to work, with modified or light duties.

Physical examination

When you have answered all the doctor's questions he will give you a physical examination. He will probably ask you to undress to your underwear in order to observe your back as you move and bend, and to feel your spine for tender areas.

Testing reflexes

The doctor will test your knee and ankle reflexes and your foot responses. He might test your leg muscles by asking you to pull your foot up while he holds it down.

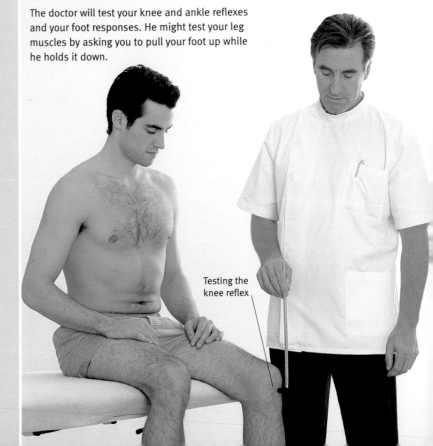

Testing the knee reflex

FURTHER TESTS

Your doctor may be more likely to investigate if the pain is very severe or prolonged or if it recurs frequently. The first tests will probably be blood tests and X-rays, though X-rays are rarely of much use in making a positive diagnosis.

A full blood count discloses the numbers of the various types of blood cell. It may reveal infection or anemia, indicating there may be an underlying disease. The ESR (erythrocyte sedimentation rate), may indicate infection, chronic inflammation, or a tumor. The ESR is usually high in inflammatory diseases of the spine, such as ankylosing spondylitis and inflammation of the sacroiliac joint.

X-rays

X-rays are only useful to exclude specific causes for the back pain, such as a fracture, spondylolysis or spondylolisthesis, a tumor, or infection, or advanced ankylosing spondylitis. The X-rays may reveal degenerative changes, including osteophyte formation (*see p. 57*) and narrowing of the disks or the foramina (the gaps between the vertebrae). However, these latter findings may not be connected with your pain.

Soft tissues, such as muscle, ligament, disk, and cartilage do not show up on X-rays. Since these tissues are usually causing the pain, X-rays often provide only negative information. In 95 percent of patients, X-rays exclude the possibility of bone

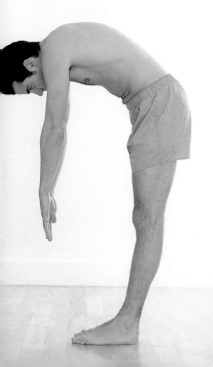

Watching your posture

The doctor will look at your posture as you stand up, and will ask you to bend forward, backward, and to each side, telling him as you do so exactly at which point the pain is worse.

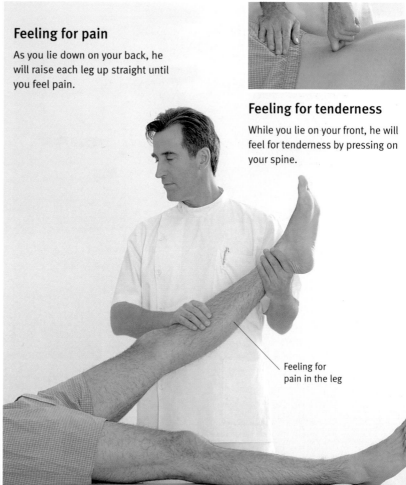

Feeling for pain

As you lie down on your back, he will raise each leg up straight until you feel pain.

Feeling for tenderness

While you lie on your front, he will feel for tenderness by pressing on your spine.

Feeling for pain in the leg

damage or serious bone disease, but do not show the real cause of the trouble. Degenerative joint disease may show up in people over 30, but this may not be causing the pain.

Consulting a specialist

If your attack is not easing after six to eight weeks of conventional treatment, and X-rays, if necessary, show either no bony cause or just simple degenerative changes, your doctor may refer you to an orthopedic, rheumatology, or physical medicine specialist.

A specialist may prefer an MRI scan to an X-ray if he feels a more specific diagnosis is required or surgery is indicated. If, however, you have been in severe pain for many weeks, have had a long time off work, and show clear signs of nerve damage to one or more of the sciatic nerves, the specialist may arrange a spinal injection for pain relief.

Further blood tests

The specialist may check the calcium, phosphate, alkaline phosphatase, and vitamin D in your blood to see if you have a bone disease. If he suspects inflammation, he may arrange an HLA-B27 test for ankylosing spondylitis.

Specialized X-rays

If you have a spinal deformity, an X-ray may help assess the angles of curvature. A curvature in the upper back may develop to compensate for a less obvious curve in the lower back. Standing X-rays may help to show if your legs are slightly different lengths or your pelvis is symmetrical.

Magnetic resonance imaging (MRI)

MRI scanning has revolutionized the investigation of the spine and musculoskeletal system and

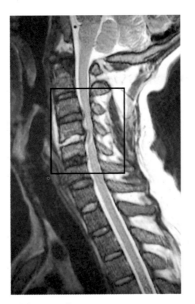

Disk protrusion
A disk that is slightly bulging is revealed in this MRI scan of a side view of the cervical spine.

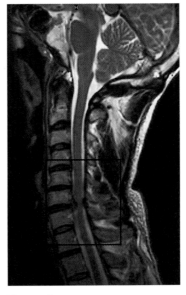

Wear and tear
This MRI scan is a side view of the cervical spine, showing the normal changes involved in wear and tear.

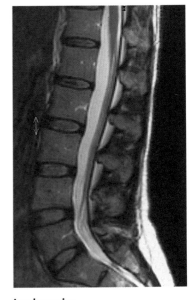

Lumbar spine
The normal lumbar spine, clearly showing the vertebrae and the disks, can be seen in this MRI scan.

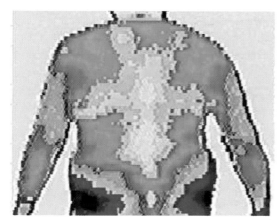

Thermograph
This colorful contour pattern of the body picks out differences in temperature as small as 0.25 °C.

have superceded myelograms. MRI scans provide a specialist with a close look at the soft tissues in and around the spine – such as disks, nerve roots, and spinal cord – which do not show up on X-rays.

As you lie on a narrow table inside a tunnel formed by a large magnet, an image is taken that is effectively a photo of a slice of your body. From a series of slices a computer can reconstruct your anatomy: muscles, ligaments, organs, and blood vessels can all be seen with brilliant clarity.

An MRI is completely noninvasive and without radiation. An MRI scan can take 30 to 40 minutes. Make sure to tell your doctor if you are worried about claustrophobia – you may be offered a sedative or, if available, an open scan.

Moire fringe analysis
Only available in a few centers in Britain, this is an excellent noninvasive way of telling whether a person's trunk symmetry – and therefore spinal balance – can be improved (for both sitting and standing).

A polarized light, shone through a diffraction grating in a darkened room, projects a contour pattern onto your back (*see right*). If the pattern is not symmetrical a lift of varying thickness is placed under one foot (or one buttock if sitting) until the best possible symmetry is obtained. Moire fringe analysis is an elegant way of answering the surprisingly complex question: is one leg shorter than the other, and if so by how much?

Thermography
This technique can demonstrate the presence of altered blood flow to the skin. A heat detector records subtle changes in skin temperature by reading the infrared waves emitted from the body (*see left*).

This technique was used in the US in the past, but it is no longer felt to have any benefit in treating patients or in monitoring changes brought about by treatment.

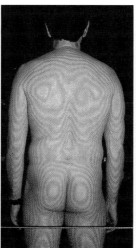
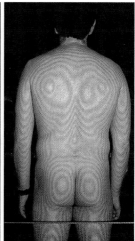

Moire fringe before
The patterns of light show that the right-hand side is clearly lower than the left.

Moire fringe after
Raising the right foot a little corrects the symmetry of the patterns.

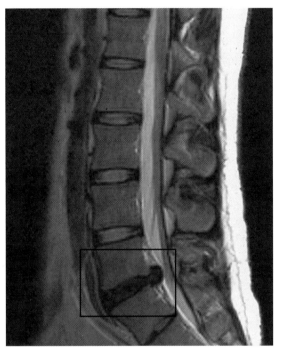

Disk protrusion
This MRI scan is a side view of the lumbar spine, showing a protruding disk at the bottom of the picture.

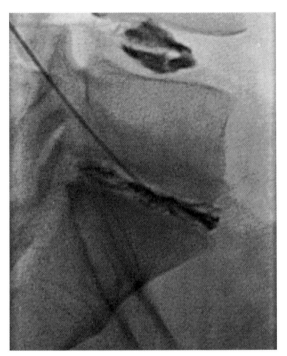

Abnormal disk
In this diskograph, the disk at the bottom (between the fifth lumbar and first sacral vertebrae) is abnormal.

CT scanning

Until the advent of MRI, this technique was widely used to investigate the spine. It shows pathological processes in bone and calcification in soft tissues better than MRI. The main disadvantage of CT scanning is that it involves higher dosages of radiation exposure than ordinary X-rays. This is because it uses an X-ray beam that goes through the body in a circular orbit to build up a cross-sectional map. Like MRI, the subject lies still in a narrow tube or tunnel for about 40 minutes.

Electromyography

This technique measures the activity of muscle groups when your spine is at rest or moving. It identifies which nerve root has been damaged, by revealing a deterioration in the activity of the muscles linked to that root. This gives more clues to locating a protruding disk. Electromyography entails inserting fine gauge needles into a muscle in the leg, foot, or calf and detecting the electrical impulses coming from it. The procedure takes about 30 minutes. There are no side effects and the only pain is a slight pricking, like a vaccination.

Diskography

This test is performed under fluoroscopy (real-time X-ray) to help identify the source of pain. After a local anesthetic, a small amount of dye is injected into the center of the disk under scrutiny. You will be asked to report the symptoms provoked by the procedure, which the investigator will compare to the usual symptoms. Diskography can identify a painful disk if an MRI has shown nothing useful.

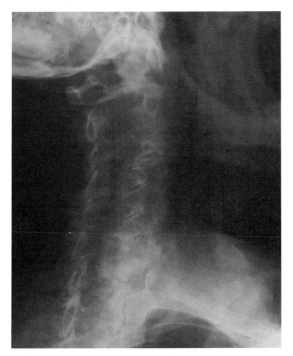

Lateral canal stenosis
This X-ray of the neck shows the narrowed foramen between the fourth and fifth cervical vertebrae.

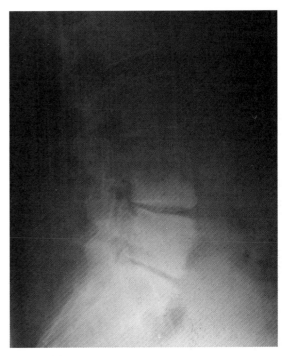

Narrow disks
This X-ray of the lumbar region shows how pressure can narrow the disks between the vertebrae.

It identifies disk disruption and is used when back or leg pain recurs after surgery for disk prolapse. It can also identify which segments are responsible for pain that can be treated by surgical fusion or less invasive techniques such as Intradiskal Electrothermal Therapy (IDET).

Facet arthrography

This technique determines whether pain in the back, hip, groin, or leg is caused by inflammation or osteoarthritis of the facet joints. It takes about 30 minutes and may be slightly painful. After a local anesthetic and under X-ray control a small amount of dye is injected into the joint to verify correct positioning. If the anesthetic relieves the symptoms, radiofrequency denervation (*see p. 105*) or a therapeutic injection can be given.

Bone scanning

A solution containing a tiny quantity of radioactive material is injected into a vein and absorbed by bone so that areas renewing themselves quickly can be identified. Increased bone turnover can be due to a variety of causes, such as a healing fracture, infection, and tumor. The pictures obtained reveal "hot spots" up to three months before they would be detected by routine X-rays. This procedure is painless and free of side effects, but it takes a couple of hours since you have to wait for the injection to take effect.

This technique has been made even more sensitive using three-dimensional imaging of the spine and by scaling up the size of the picture to give a color differential picture – a SPECT scan – showing the precise site of abnormal bone activity.

5

Manipulation

An increasing number of doctors now offer manipulation as a viable alternative to conventional treatment for low back pain, and more and more people are seeking manipulative therapy from a physical therapist. The treatment involves the manual adjustment of the joints in the spine and is beneficial to a variety of spinal disorders.

The medical manipulation practiced by some doctors and physical therapists is not significantly different from the techniques employed by osteopaths and chiropractors, except that it is more

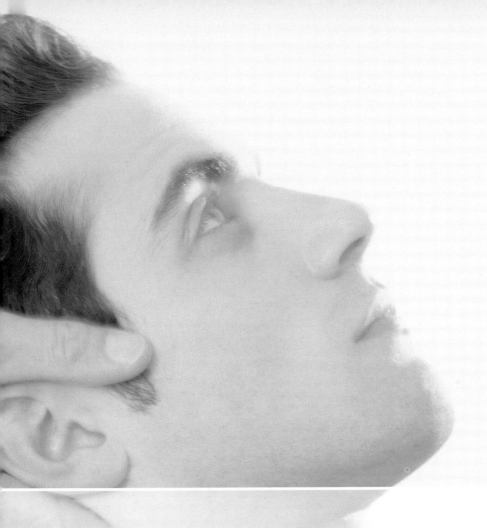

likely to include traction when treating the neck. The major
distinction is that doctors attempt to make a medical diagnosis
before starting treatment, and then concentrate on resolving that
particular problem. Osteopaths and chiropractors often treat simply
by feeling which spinal segment is at fault. They may approach the
problem indirectly and continue treatment after the symptoms have
disappeared. The three case histories in this chapter demonstrate the
different techniques used.

Approaches to treating back pain

The differences between chiropractic and medical manipulation (physical therapy) are best shown by describing a typical treatment for each. These reveal the benefits of manipulative treatment for both acute and chronic problems, even if the symptoms are not confined to the spine.

MANIPULATION: MINOR DISK PROTRUSION

Manipulation is of value for various back disorders, even when the pain may be referred and appears to come from a different source.

Symptoms

Joanne, a 20-year-old engineering student, consulted an osteopath about an acute attack of pain in her right hip and the region of her groin. She had been studying intensively for her exams, which meant that she was spending long hours in front of her computer in a less than ideal posture.

For several weeks Joanne had been experiencing pain in her right hip and in her lower abdomen toward the groin. After sitting for too long she had difficulty in standing straight, due to the pain in the groin. After a while Joanne could walk normally and the pain would lessen. A cough or sneeze seemed to hurt in the groin.

Treatment by manipulation

The doctor rotated Joanne's spine carefully using a rotation with distraction technique – in other words, rotating the spine while simultaneously easing the joints open on one side. He then asked Joanne to stand up and checked her movements again. Only bending forward was painful this time. The doctor then applied a second manipulation with Joanne lying face down, and again checked her ability to move.

Stretching the right side

The doctor put one hand on Joanne's right shoulder and the other on her right hip. While pushing her shoulder and hip down to rotate her spine, he leaned forward, letting his body weight stretch Joanne's right side.

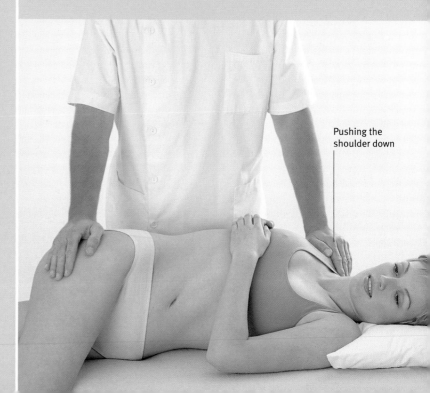

Pushing the shoulder down

Examination

The doctor took a case history and discovered that Joanne had been experiencing some menstrual irregularity, including vaginal discharge and painful periods.

The doctor performed a thorough physical examination. He asked Joanne to bend forward, backward, and to each side, in order to check the flexibility of her spine. Joanne's movement was restricted in two directions and her groin ached when she tried to bend too far.

Then, with Joanne lying on her front, the doctor felt each individual spinal segment. He discovered that her spine was particularly sensitive to pressure between the fourth and fifth lumbar vertebrae.

During his investigation he conducted a pelvic examination, as well as a pap smear and swab to check for infection. He also palpated her abdomen and checked for hernia in the groin. He carefully assessed Joanne's hip joints for restriction or pain. The results of the tests were normal.

Diagnosis

The doctor suspected that Joanne had a minor disk protrusion, which bulged to the right, between the fourth and fifth lumbar vertebrae, referring pain to the hip and groin. In addition, he suspected that the sacroiliac ligaments in Joanne's lower back were strained, since she showed signs of excessive mobility in the sacroiliac joints.

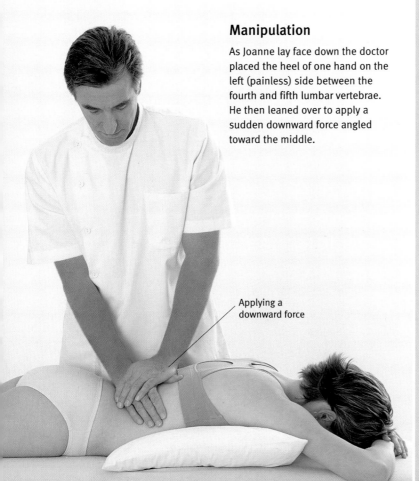

Applying a
downward force

Manipulation

As Joanne lay face down the doctor placed the heel of one hand on the left (painless) side between the fourth and fifth lumbar vertebrae. He then leaned over to apply a sudden downward force angled toward the middle.

Recovery

After two treatments, Joanne recovered her full range of movement. The doctor advised her on posture and regular exercise. She was offered prolotherapy (*see p. 101*) in order to stabilize the affected sacroiliac joints.

OSTEOPATHY: ACUTE LUMBAGO

This is a fairly typical case of acute lower back pain, which is brought on by awkward twisting and bending of the spine.

Symptoms

Joanne had been experiencing an intermittent mild ache in her lower back for some time, usually after driving, but it lasted only a few hours. However, during a game of tennis she felt a sudden very sharp pain in her lower back, which eased to a dull ache for the rest of the day.

The next morning, the pain was piercing again and shot down her right leg. Certain movements made it worse – bending backward and to the right were particularly painful, so Joanne adopted a position slightly bent forward and leaning to the left. Joanne decided this time to consult an osteopath to deal with the acute pain.

Examination

The osteopath made a diagnosis through physical examination, asking Joanne to bend her back and describe the pain this provoked. Bending slightly to the right, she had sharp pain in the back and down the right leg. If she bent backward, she felt severe pain across her lower back. However, bending forward or to the left did not hurt her.

The osteopath asked Joanne to lie down on her back, and then lifted each of her legs. The left

Treatment by an osteopath

The osteopath first massaged Joanne's back to relax the muscles. The massage also stretched the spine slightly, which helped to reduce pressure on the disk. After about five minutes Joanne could lie comfortably without cushions, the pain in her leg had receded and the back pain was more central. Then the osteopath manipulated the spinal segments to encourage the disk protrusion to recede.

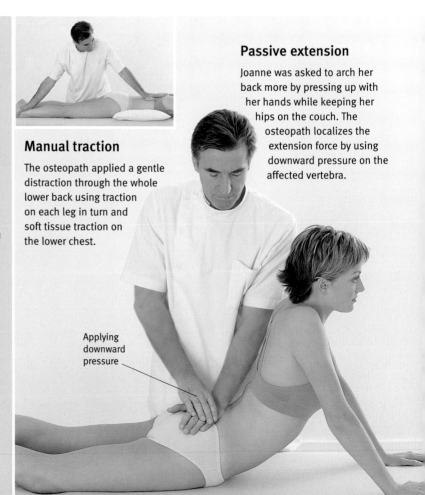

Manual traction

The osteopath applied a gentle distraction through the whole lower back using traction on each leg in turn and soft tissue traction on the lower chest.

Passive extension

Joanne was asked to arch her back more by pressing up with her hands while keeping her hips on the couch. The osteopath localizes the extension force by using downward pressure on the affected vertebra.

Applying downward pressure

could be raised to about 60° before it was painful, but raising the right leg caused the same piercing pain. Lying on her front was painful, since this arched her lower back slightly. But with cushions under her stomach, which had the effect of making her lower spine flat, Joanne could lie comfortably without feeling pain.

Diagnosis

From this examination, the osteopath diagnosed that Joanne was suffering from a protruding disk. It was bulging to the right and pressing against the sciatic nerve. Since Joanne was comfortable lying down with her spine straight, the osteopath deduced that the disk was not fixed in its new

position. As a consequence, the disk might be reducible as soon as the upper part of the spine was not pressing on it. This suggested that gentle manipulation combined with manual traction would be sufficient to cure the problem.

CHIROPRACTOR: WHIPLASH

This example shows how manipulation of spinal joints by a chiropractor can help problems that are not always associated with spinal disorders.

Symptoms

Mike approached a chiropractor for help because he has been suffering from headaches that were accompanied with pain and stiffness in both

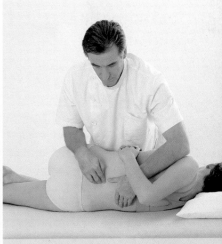

Rotational manipulation

As Joanne lay on her front, the osteopath mobilized the lower lumbar segments in turn by applying a firm pressure at the side of each vertebra with his thumb and gently rotating and abducting the leg.

Rotating and abducting the leg

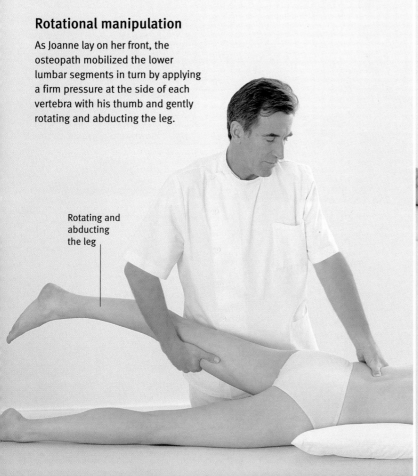

Recovery

After this treatment, Joanne no longer had pain in her leg and she could stand straight and bend backward. The osteopath instructed her to rest for a few days and to repeat the passive extension exercise twice a day. A few days later Joanne returned for a more specific manipulation using leverage (*above*).

his neck and his back. He was also complaining of intermittent pins and needles down his right arm into his thumb and index finger.

Examination

The chiropractor took a full medical history and discovered that Mike had been experiencing these symptoms since suffering a whiplash injury in a car accident three years earlier. He had not been X-rayed at that time, nor had he been ill since. He had been taking pain medication for the headaches.

The chiropractor checked Mike's blood pressure and tested the reflexes of his arm muscles. He checked that the pupils of his eyes could contract and dilate properly. His blood pressure and eye reflexes were normal, but the reflexes in his right arm were slightly slower than those in his left arm. The chiropractor rotated and extended Mike's neck to determine whether the vertebral artery, which supplies blood to the brain, was constricted. However, it was normal.

Finally, the chiropractor examined Mike's spine for its ability to twist and bend. Mike could twist his head to the left easily and without pain, but his neck was stiff and painful when he tried to turn to the right. Bending his head forward caused him pain in his midback.

The greatest stiffness was between the second and third cervical vertebrae. Mike's thoracic spine was examined as he lay face down on a couch.

Treatment by a chiropractor

Chiropractors have specially designed couches divided into four sections, which can be raised or lowered independently of each other. This enables a chiropractor to use sharp thrusting movements to manipulate the spine.

By lowering the appropriate section of the couch at the moment he thrusts down on a vertebra, the chiropractor can increase the movement of one segment of the back while minimizing the force on the spine.

The chiropractor treated two vertebrae in Mike's back in this way, checking the mobility of his back and neck each time.

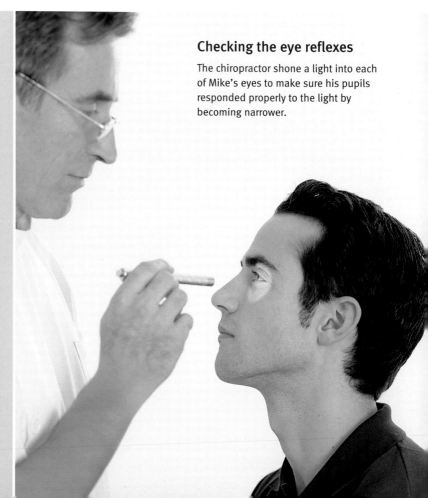

Checking the eye reflexes

The chiropractor shone a light into each of Mike's eyes to make sure his pupils responded properly to the light by becoming narrower.

The chiropractor felt each joint individually and discovered that there was a slight stiffness in Mike's midback between the sixth and seventh thoracic vertebrae.

Diagnosis

The chiropractor diagnosed that the whiplash injury had resulted in stiffness between the second and third vertebrae in Mike's neck and between the sixth and seventh thoracic vertebrae. This lack of mobility, or perhaps fibrous tissue from the accident, prevented the nerves in these area from functioning properly. This explained Mike's pins and needles, as well as the sluggish reflex in his right arm and the headaches.

Consulting a physical therapist

A physical therapist makes a thorough assessment of the spine and its related functions before starting treatment. Diagnosis starts from the moment you walk into the room. The physical therapist takes a full history of your symptoms and then examines you to assess the way you move. He observes the way you walk, stand, and sit, and will then ask you to bend forward, backward, and sideways.

His preliminary examination is very similar to the doctor's (*see p. 76*). He will also feel your back,

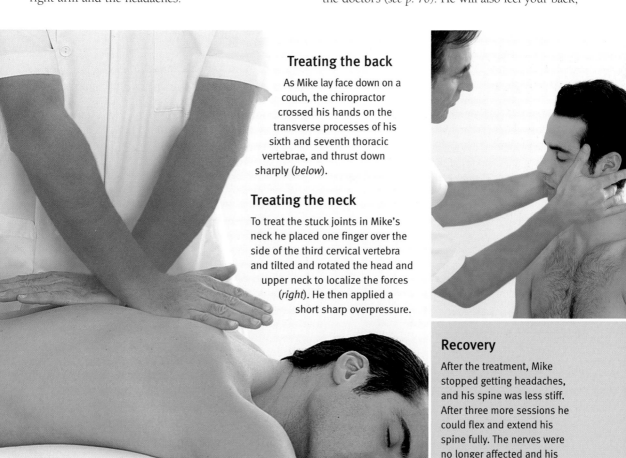

Treating the back

As Mike lay face down on a couch, the chiropractor crossed his hands on the transverse processes of his sixth and seventh thoracic vertebrae, and thrust down sharply (*below*).

Treating the neck

To treat the stuck joints in Mike's neck he placed one finger over the side of the third cervical vertebra and tilted and rotated the head and upper neck to localize the forces (*right*). He then applied a short sharp overpressure.

Recovery

After the treatment, Mike stopped getting headaches, and his spine was less stiff. After three more sessions he could flex and extend his spine fully. The nerves were no longer affected and his symptoms disappeared.

testing the movement of individual segments, and feeling for tender or tense spots in the muscles.

PRELIMINARY TREATMENT

A physical therapist's tools are his hands: he is trained in a variety of methods of manipulation and massage, though techniques may differ between therapists. The Maitlands method (*see below*) is one of the most common techniques. The physical therapist may also use electrotherapy equipment such as ultrasound.

Massage

This is more than just a pleasurable, relaxing ancillary treatment. It can be therapeutic when applied to taut muscles and, since it relaxes you, it is an important preliminary to manipulation.

Massage given by a physical therapist is likely to include deep transverse friction massage. The therapist massages with his fingers across the fibers of ligaments and muscles to break up scar tissue, improve blood supply, and increase mobility. He may use connective tissue massage, a technique that involves stretching the skin by drawing the fingertip over certain pathways to stimulate blood flow and encourage the muscles to relax.

Other methods of massage include stroking, kneading, vibratory movements, and petrissage (pinching and stretching adjacent muscle areas), which all help to reduce fluid in the muscle tissue.

Maitlands mobilization

All physical therapists in Britain, and some in the US, learn and use the Maitlands method to mobilize spinal and other joints. This entails gentle rhythmic movements of a spinal joint near the limit of its normal range of movement. Sometimes a thrust is made beyond the normal "joint range," but only with your consent and not to cause pain.

Ultrasound

One of physical therapy's most popular therapeutic tools, ultrasound treats soft tissue injuries, such as damage to a muscle, ligament, tendon, or joint capsule. It can be used for trigger points (*see p. 48*) – it encourages the localized contractions of the muscles to relax – and for treating injured muscles. Studies suggest that the high-frequency sound waves promote healing by speeding up the different phases of the inflammatory and repair processes in the affected body cells.

Ultrasound is very popular in sports injuries centers and can be used to drive a solution of anti-inflammatory cream or cortisone through the skin to settle inflammation in the soft tissues or joints.

You receive the treatment on a couch with the relevant part of your back exposed. It is normally entirely painless without any sensation. Relief from pain is not immediate and it is normal to have two or three sessions a week over a few weeks.

Shortwave diathermy

High-frequency electromagnetic waves are used to promote a healing action in the tissues. It reduces swelling, stabilizes cell membranes, and stimulates blood flow, and so results in muscle relaxation, decreased joint stiffness, and a reduction of pain. To prevent the tissues from overheating, the waves can be given as pulses, which allows the tissues to cool down between doses. Shortwave diathermy has been used to heal nonunited fractures, suggesting that its effects are more far-reaching than those of straightforward heat treatment.

You lie on a couch with the relevant part of your back exposed. The treatment is painless and you feel better immediately, but you will probably need two or three treatments a week for several weeks. There are no side effects since the machines automatically give out a pulsed wave which has no deep heating effect. This allows treatment to be given soon after the injury, even if there is still some local bleeding.

Electrical stimulation

This is another form of electrotherapy in which a low frequency "interference" wave is produced where two medium frequency alternating currents coincide. The therapist can vary the frequency of the wave according to which tissue – nerves, muscles, or blood vessels – he wants to influence. This therapy helps reduce inflammation in joints or muscles.

Electrical stimulation may be applied through damp sponges covering electrodes or via suction caps. You experience a "fizzy" sensation from the electric current and your muscles may twitch involuntarily if the lower frequency ranges are used. There are no known side effects. The pain relief may be immediate but often lasts only a short time so you need two or three sessions a week for a few weeks. However, there is little evidence as to the treatment's long-term value.

Transcutaneous nerve stimulation

This treatment is used by physical therapists and pain clinics throughout the world to help people suffering severe pain (*see p. 169*).

TRACTION

This method of treatment is declining due to a lack of evidence for its efficacy. Traction is used to pull the spinal joints apart very gently, enabling the muscles in the back to relax fully, and reducing pressure within the disk. The stretching relieves facet joints that have been compressed by the weight of your body when you stand up. All this may relieve pain and even accelerate recovery.

If traction is applied properly, using chest and pelvic harnesses on a lumbar traction table, the only discomfort you may experience will be due to the tightness of the harnesses. However, if you have been in traction for 20 minutes or so, you might feel painful twinges as it is being released. If you experience pain as traction is being put on and increased, tell the therapist to stop immediately. This may indicate that the protrusion is being pushed harder against the nerve root, particularly if the pain is worse in your leg, and traction is therefore an inappropriate form of treatment for you.

Traction is best given daily to let its cumulative effects accelerate recovery. You may feel immediate pain relief, and although the pain might return partially or even completely, it will be reduced by subsequent treatments. Alternatively, it may be a week before you begin to feel any benefit. If your condition does not improve after two weeks, this therapy is unlikely to bring you relief.

Inversion therapy

Of the new variations on the theme of traction, inversion therapy looks the most natural and promising. Inversion therapy is useful in a similar range of back conditions to those treated by horizontal traction.

Various machines enable you to treat yourself at home or at work simply by strapping your ankles to a tilt frame and swinging backward – literally turning you upside down. If your doctor or physical therapist decides that it would be right for you, he will supervise the first one or two sessions and, if there is no complication, you may well be able to take the apparatus home and use it at your convenience.

Since back pain is characteristically a recurring problem and the disk degenerates with age, there is a case for recommending the use of a portable inversion traction machine on a regular basis – say, 10 to 15 minutes a day – at home.

Once you are accustomed to the blood rushing to your head, inversion traction feels comfortable. Unlike horizontal traction, there are no tight harnesses restricting your breathing or circulation. You can operate the machine yourself simply by moving your arms and you can use it as often as you like, when you like, in your own home.

Muscles relax quite quickly in the fully inverted position, and the length of the spine measurably increases after only a few minutes. Some of this lengthening effect may be attributed to a certain amount of reabsorption of fluid into the center of the disk, which nourishes the disk cartilage. Used over a long period, this inversion therapy may

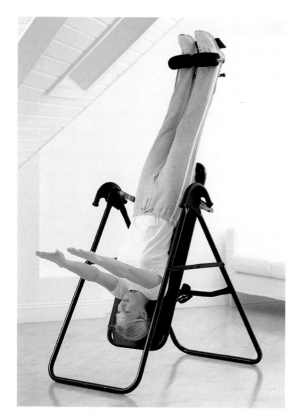

Inversion therapy
10 to 15 minutes a day on an inversion traction machine can help back muscles relax.

delay the degenerative process that occurs due to "drying out," though so far there is no firm evidence to prove this theory. The remaining effect is probably due to improved posture. Inversion therapy may also aid the drainage of the veins in the spinal canal, reducing congestion and helping to speed up the healing process.

Although the treatment is completely safe, if you do not suffer from high blood pressure, a history of strokes, or glaucoma (high pressure in the eyeball), I would not advise anyone to invest in this equipment before consulting their doctor.

COLLARS AND CORSETS

A painful back or neck may need extra support, so a therapist may give you a collar or a corset to wear temporarily. Whether it can relieve acute pain or speed up your recovery is in dispute.

A corset reduces the pressure on your spine by supporting your abdomen; it is supposed to restrict movement but some research suggests that your lower spine bends even more if you wear a corset which comes high up your back. A collar helps support your head and therefore reduces the pressure on your neck.

A collar or corset can also provide warmth and stimulate the pressure-sensitive nerve endings in the skin – an effect similar to massage. A collar or corset reminds you to be careful of how you move or bend. It may help your muscles to relax and may provide short-term relief.

Cervical collars

Collars are less frequently employed to relieve an acutely painful neck condition than they once were. This is largely because there is mounting evidence to suggest that, by using a cervical collar, a patient is not only afraid of moving but also becomes dependent on the collar for support. Whether your painful neck

Collars and corsets

Collars are either made of foam or rigid plastic. Most corsets are made from a combination of canvas and elastic, foam, or neoprene, depending on the amount of flexibility they are intended to provide. There are various kinds of corset – short, long, light and flexible, heavy and ribbed, with or without thoracic bands, lateral uprights, and sacral extensions – and a range of sizes to use "off the shelf." A more rigid corset can be made especially to suit your body's particular needs.

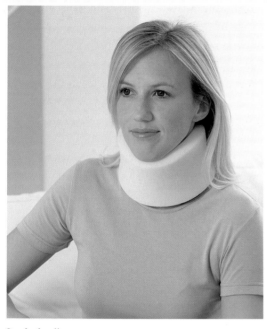

Cervical collar
This soft collar supports the head, takes weight off the neck, and restricts neck movement. They are only a temporary measure and should not be worn for too long.

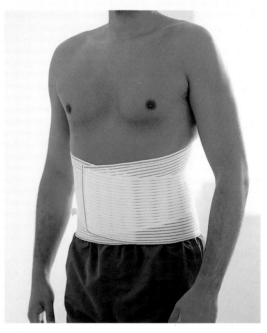

Spinal corset
It is important that a corset fits exactly, in order to support the spine while allowing you to sit comfortably. If you need one for long-term use it can be tailored to your shape.

has developed suddenly on waking one morning, or is the result of a whiplash injury, a supportive cervical collar may help to relieve the pain. It works by restricting your neck movements and providing support for your head. A cervical collar is only a temporary measure to allow the inflammation or bruising around the spinal joints to settle down. You may not need to wear the collar all the time, and you probably will not have to use it for more than a few days.

A condition that is more likely to benefit from a collar is vertebro-basilar syndrome. The vertebral artery, which travels up the neck through a bony canal created on either side of the vertebrae, may be narrowed or compressed in certain positions when you turn your head or stretch your neck. This brings on sudden dizziness and occasionally blackouts when you look up, turn around, or work with your arms held up – for example, hanging laundry or painting a ceiling. The vertebro-basilar syndrome is partly an effect of the narrowing and hardening of the arteries which tend to occur with age. People with these symptoms, should see a doctor. Those who suffer from this generalized disease of the circulation, combined with narrowing of the vertebral artery, may need to control the symptoms by wearing a hard collar all the time to restrict neck movements.

Corsets

Today, spinal corsets are used much less frequently than they once were. Physical therapists tend to recommend wearing a corset only as a short-term measure, perhaps for a few weeks after recovering from an acute episode of back pain to enable you to go back to work without risking an early relapse. Very few people are in favor of any long-term use of corsets because your spinal joints may become stiff.

OTHER TREATMENTS

The physical therapist will probably advise you on posture and lifting and handling techniques (*see pp. 148–149*). He may also recommend a course on back care (*see Functional rehabilitation, right*) and teach you some therapeutic exercises (*see Chapter 7*). Some types of back pain can be eased and relieved by performing gentle stretching and bending exercises in warm water (*see Hydrotherapy, below*). General fitness training is increasingly advocated to improve endurance capacity.

Hydrotherapy

Traditionally, the wealthy sought relief from pain in health spas with warm water springs or special minerals. The common factor in these hydrotherapy treatments is the weightless effect of floating in water; what goes into the water – salt, mud, or sulphur – is probably of minor importance.

Most large hospital physical therapy departments and well-supplied private clinics have a pool for supervised treatment of many forms of muscle and joint injury. You can do exercises to strengthen and stretch muscles, while the water supports you and reduces pressure on your joints.

Flexibility and mobility can both be achieved without the risk of exceeding the "normal" range of movement, because the resistance offered by the water restricts your actions. Swimming, too, can have a definite therapeutic effect as long as you do not arch your back while doing the breast stroke in an attempt to keep your head above water.

Functional rehabilitation

First developed in Sweden about 30 years ago, the Back School approach is used in varying forms by a growing number of physical therapy departments in Britain, Europe, the United States, and Australia. Functional rehabilitation is not appropriate if you are suffering an episode of acute back pain because its purpose is to help those with a long-term back problem.

A variety of rehabilitation programs are available, focusing on the needs of different groups of patients. Every program differs but the main forms of treatment are:

• Postural advice – in standing, sitting, and lying.
• Specific muscle strengthening exercises for the muscles of the abdomen, back, and legs.
• Hydrotherapy.
• Education – the mechanics of the spine, including its anatomy and its physiology; lifting and handling techniques;
• Ergonomics, including choosing equipment, tools, furniture, and the shape, size, and weight of loads to minimize strain on the spine.
• Confidence building.
• General fitness training.

The main benefit of attending a rehabilitation program is its comprehensive approach to all the factors. You will be offered: a thorough clinical examination; a functional assessment to see how you manage everyday tasks; appropriate therapeutic treatment; and group classes. The program is combined with follow-up treatment and support from a team of experts, which may include orthopedic specialists, psychologists, and specialists in vocational rehabilitation.

Studies of the effectiveness of functional rehabilitation programs have shown that symptoms tend to clear up sooner and that less time is lost from work. Participants often increase the amount of exercise they subsequently get and become less dependent on passive treatment approaches to back pain.

Osteopathy

An osteopathic physician's training is similar to that of a MD physician. However, osteopaths receive additional training in manipulation. Increasing numbers of MD physicians, however, are now practicing manipulation. An osteopath emphasizes function – that is, abnormal movement of the joint is the essential feature in a spinal disorder. He tends to use more indirect than direct leverage, and often employs a rhythmic stretching of the ligaments around the joint to restore the optimal range of movement. His techniques are aimed at loosening and freeing rather than at repositioning.

Chiropractic

Although chiropractors have increasingly tended to conform to basic medical training, most retain a holistic approach to the patient. Chiropractors view back pain in the context of disorders of the whole spine, pelvis, lower limbs, and muscle imbalance. These therapists may also give advice on diet – a factor which conventional doctors might not link to back pain.

Chiropractors recognize that structure and function cannot be separated. A chiropractor is perhaps more likely to see the problem in terms of the spine's structure, in particular the position of the bones. For this reason his treatment is aimed at repositioning specific bones using thrusting techniques.

Consulting a practitioner

If manipulation has helped to relieve your back pain in the past, and the problem recurs, it may help you again and should be considered.

However, manipulation may be of no value in some conditions, and can even be dangerous. For this reason, it is wise to inform your primary care doctor before seeking any manipulation and also why your chiropractor must know what is wrong with you – at least in general terms – before you have manipulation.

Very occasionally, back pain can be a symptom of cancer, for example, in which case manipulation is inappropriate and could be dangerous. In inflammatory conditions such as ankylosing spondylitis, where the spinal ligaments calcify to lock the spine rigid, manipulation is of no use, though not actually dangerous. A well-qualified and conscientious manipulator will discriminate between those patients who will and those who will not benefit from manipulation.

Each practitioner, whether medically qualified or not, varies in his approach. Most will ask questions and examine you in a similar way and may include some other methods of examination according to his own preference.

Relieving pain

If you are considering whether to consult a chiropractor, you will probably want to know whether he can alleviate your back pain. Unfortunately, it is impossible to give a definite answer. This is because no two cases are identical – even relatively slight differences of age, weight, fitness, or will to recover can affect the success of nonmedical manipulation. So, too, can the rapport between therapist and patient. Whether you are referred to a practitioner by your doctor or whether you approach one directly, it is important that you are able to get along well with the therapist and you feel you can him. If you are going to benefit from treatment, you will probably feel some relief from pain after two or three sessions. If the pain is unchanged, your condition is unlikely to improve with further sessions.

Conditions that may respond to manipulation

Manipulation may be offered as a preventative technique to keep the spine mobile. Claims that it delays degenerative changes (*see p. 56*), or prevents acute problems such as "stuck" facet joints (*see pp. 43–44*), remain to be proven.

If muscles have been weakened because a nerve has been pinched, manipulation can free the nerve, which allows both strength and movement to be restored. Manipulation may also help conditions such as migraines, premenstrual tension, and constipation, via reflex effects.

The back conditions listed below are most likely to respond to, and benefit from, treatment by a manipulative therapist.

Braces and casts for structural scoliosis

Nonsurgical treatment of scoliosis depends on the amount of curvature. If the curve is very slight, causing no discomfort and minimal deformity, then it may not be necessary to treat the condition.

Exercises (*see Chapter 7*) improve flexibility and posture but they do not prevent the development of the curve. They are helpful in mild scoliosis as well as in the slightly more severe cases that need braces. Exercises may also be recommended to increase flexibility before surgery.

Braces are commonly used to treat more pronounced curves. A Milwaukee brace, for example, can help patients whose lumbar spine curves to the left, while the thoracic spine curves to the right. To correct the thoracic curve, a pad over the right shoulder blade is counteracted by a sling under the left arm. A pad fitted over the left side of the waist should be able to straighten the lumbar spine.

A "low profile" brace is equipped with pads on the inside that are positioned to correct the curve of the spine.

Supports for the shoulders can be attached to the brace if the spine is also rotated.

Braces are prescribed and fitted by orthotists. They are normally worn for 23 hours a day and removed only for bathing or recommended exercises. Once growing has stopped or the curve has improved, braces can be worn for more reduced periods of time.

Babies with scoliosis may be put into plaster cast braces with pressure pads inside and a window cut in the concave side to allow the ribs to grow normally.

Neck pain

In acute cases of torticollis (*see p. 38*), which is often caused by sleeping in an awkward position, manipulation has a limited application. Massage can relax taut muscles and gentle traction can restore movement. If the capsule around the joint is overstretched and inflamed so that moving it is painful, the practitioner will apply traction very carefully, and then place your head and neck as close as possible to the normal resting position. He will repeat this process every ten minutes.

Osteoarthritis

Gentle manipulation can help when this disease affects the lumbar vertebrae. Some help can be given to maintain mobility but none can relieve the inflammation of the joints.

Disk prolapse

If you have severe lumbago, the practitioner will help you find the most comfortable resting position. He may even bring relief with gentle manual traction. After a few days' rest, your pain may have subsided enough for you to have some very gentle manipulation.

Sciatica

Manipulation may be help if a disk protrusion is causing pain in the leg, but only if there are no signs of nerve damage. Even so, the therapist may help you find a pain-relieving position.

Chronic muscular tension

If you are suffering from chronic muscular tension, manipulation of the joints can help to relax them, but only temporarily. The practitioner, however, may stretch the muscles rhythmically and advise you on appropriate exercises to strengthen your muscles without straining them (*see Chapter 7*).

Sacroiliac strain

Manipulation can align the iliac bone and the sacrum properly and ease the strain, but too much manipulation can stretch the ligaments and make the condition worse.

Facet joint dysfunction

Manipulation can help to free facet joints that have become strained or stuck. Manual traction can is useful for disk or facet joint problems that have resulted from a whiplash injury if it is applied soon after the pain and stiffness started.

Rib lesions

When the head of a rib, where it is attached to a vertebra, is either elevated or depressed, manipulation can restore the correct position.

Functional scoliosis

If you have scoliosis, a condition in which the spine is curved over to one side, the success of manipulation depends on various factors. If X-rays show that the shape of the vertebrae is normal, you may be leaning over to one side to minimize pain that is caused, perhaps, by a disk protrusion. This is known as functional scoliosis, and manipulation may help to cure the underlying cause. However, if X-rays show that you have structural scoliosis (*see p. 54*), in which one side of the vertebra is narrower than the other, manipulation can not help .

 If one leg is longer than the other, the pelvis may tilt, which produces changes in posture. It is easy to correct the leg length simply by raising the height of one shoe. This corrects the sideways tilt of the pelvis and over time gradually reforms the curve farther up the spine. However, there is a risk that this might also cause more aches and pains than the adapted posture.

6

Drugs and Surgery

Back pain is caused by many factors so a doctor, who combines advice, drugs, or injections, may well be acting on sound holistic principles. It is perfectly possible, for example, that muscle relaxants, pain medication, and modified activity are the best way to put you into the optimum mental and physical state for the healing process to begin.

Only a tiny minority of people with back problems need surgery. If your doctor suggests an operation you will probably have already tried several other treatments unsuccessfully. Surgery is the only way

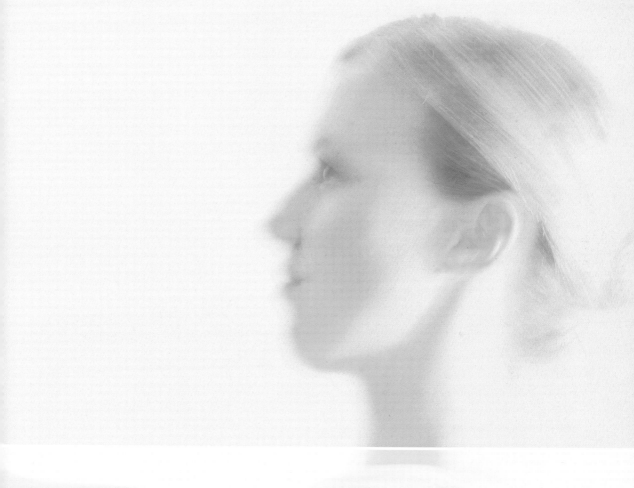

to deal with certain kinds of bone infections and tumors. If your spine is still very painful and other treatments have failed to correct the problem, you will need to undergo some specialized tests, such as MRI scans, diskography, and CT scans (*see Chapter 4*). These will reveal whether your condition could be helped with an operation. The most common reason for spinal surgery is to treat disk problems. A small proportion of surgery is done to stabilize fractures or other segments of the spine where nerves are compressed and damaged.

Treatment with drugs

Doctors use a wide range of drugs to relieve and cure back pain, from simple over-the-counter pain medication to drugs for specific conditions.

Simple pain medication

Pain medication, such as codeine, aspirin, and acetaminophen, are available over the counter and are useful for managing mild to moderate pain.

Combination drugs

Acetaminophen, or aspirin, ibuprofen or codeine combined with another drug, can relieve mild to moderate pain.Some of these combination drugs are also available over the counter.

Strong analgesics

These include narcotics such as morphine and meperidine, and nonnarcotic opioids such as tramadol. If you are in severe pain, unable to find comfort in any position, and unable to sleep, you need strong pain medication, particularly if your pain continues for more than 12 to 24 hours.

Nonnarcotics have few side effects, but are often less effective than narcotics. However, the latter may cause constipation and drowsiness. Many doctors are reluctant to prescribe strong narcotics for fear patients may become addicted. In short-term acute pain this is an unnecessary fear; even long-term use is unlikely to result in dependency. But evidence suggests that some people are naturally prone to addiction. If you are worried about this, discuss it with your doctor.

If you suffer from severe lumbar or cervical radiculopathy caused by nerve root compression, it is my belief that good pain relief in the early stages will help prevent the sort of sensitization to pain which can delay recovery.

Muscle relaxants

In acute neck pain or lower back pain, when the muscles tend to tighten up to protect the painful area from further injury, muscle relaxants can help. If you are high strung or apprehensive, your muscles may stay tense longer than necessary after the injury and can remain fixed like this even after the injury has started to heal.

Massage or relaxation therapy may help; or you may be given diazepam or similar for two or three days. The drawback to this is that it will slow you down mentally and make you drowsy, and long-term use can lead to dependency. Unfortunately, muscle relaxants are all too often prescribed for people who have no real need for them.

Anti-inflammatory drugs

Many doctors now prescribe these routinely for all musculoskeletal pain to treat joints that become painful. They are the mainstay of drug treatment of back pain in the US. Their advantage is through the anti-inflammatory effect, which plays an important role in easing pain. Common side effects include nausea, gastric irritation, and the occasional internal hemorrhage. Even the newer varieties of anti-inflammatory drugs still do not offer better relief from pain and stiffness than standard drugs such as codeine.

Steroids

These synthetic drugs are very similar to the body's natural steroid hormones. They are prescribed in much larger quantities than the body is used to, and they work by a powerful anti-inflammatory action. Corticosteroids can help some of the conditions that affect all the joints of the body, including the spine.

Long-term oral steroids have side effects such as weight gain, acne, hairiness, diabetes, high blood pressure, reduced resistance to infection, and osteoporosis. However, a much smaller quantity of corticosteroid, given in a local injection to reduce swelling and irritation around a nerve root or to treat inflammation in a joint, probably has minimal side effects.

Drugs for osteoporosis

If your bones have degenerated severely and become thin and brittle, some mineral and vitamin supplements can help strengthen them or slow down the rate of mineral loss. Calcium and vitamin D may build up the bones again, and new drugs called bisphosphonates are extremely effective in preventing vertebral compression fractures.

Injections

Injections are a marvelously accurate and effective way of delivering treatment to the specific source of trouble. Why take a general and nonspecific course of treatment when a local, specific treatment with low risk of side effects can be given? But do not expect immediate relief – it may take a few days before your back pain begins to recede. The success of the treatment also depends to some extent on you following your doctor's advice on how to look after your back, both between treatments and after the course.

MUSCULAR INJECTIONS

Trigger points (*see p. 48*) are often successfully treated with a course of local injections containing a small dose of local anesthetic, unless the joints nearby are the source of the problem. If this is the case, the joints themselves have to be treated first, and the muscles should then relax of their own accord. Local injections are often most helpful if they are combined with stretching exercises and a cooling spray to help muscles relax. The treatment can be given in your doctor's office.

LIGAMENT INJECTIONS

If your pain comes from sprained ligaments, you might find that the injury is slow to heal. A few people need a local injection of steroid combined with some local anesthetic.

Procedure

The doctor will identify your strained ligament with his fingers and inject a drop of steroid at one end and, shifting the needle slightly each time, inject the ligament along its length and breadth. You may experience some soreness or aching for 24 to 48 hours. You need to refrain from excessive lifting, carrying, and bending, and avoid sitting in one position for long periods.

You need to take it easy because the steroid injection weakens the collagen fiber that provides tension in the ligaments. After 10 to 14 days, the collagen returns to normal and your doctor will see you again to assess progress.

PROLOTHERAPY

Chronic ligament strain, particularly in the lower back and sacroiliac joints, is common in people whose backs feel unstable. This feeling could be due, for example, to narrow disks causing the facet joints to cram together, or perhaps to a recurrent strain of the sacroiliac joint.

Normal mobility can be restored by injecting sclerosant into the ligaments which control the motion of the relevant segment or joint. This treatment is also helpful in mild spondylolisthesis, when one vertebra shifts slightly. Tighter ligaments help to hold the vertebra more securely in position.

Sclerosant injections contain a small amount of fibrous tissue irritant (phenol and dextrose) in an inert solution such as glycerine. The sclerosant stimulates the production of fibrous tissue and new collagen, and after several injections at weekly intervals the ligament becomes thicker and even stronger where the ligament and bone meet.

Procedure

If your lower back is to be treated, you will lie on your front over a pillow or cushion so that your lower back region is slightly rounded (*see below*). The sclerosant is mixed with a local anesthetic to dull the initial burning pain.

The procedure can be painful but takes only 10 to 15 minutes. You may be given gas and air to help you relax, and some practitioners prefer you to be under a general anesthetic. When the local anesthetic has worn off after an hour, there is a sensation of bruising. This may last for two or three days and is due to your ligaments reacting to the fibrous tissue irritant. There are rarely any other side effects.

Most physicians use a course of three weekly injections. Keep bending or lifting to a minimum during the next three weeks. In the fourth and fifth weeks after the treatment you should walk three miles (five kilometers) each day to encourage

Prolotherapy

The doctor will be able to locate the position of the ligaments by feeling for the top of your iliac bone on each side and the spinous processes of your lumbar vertebrae. He will then draw a grid on your back using these bones as reference points to help him position the needle in exactly the right place. Even if the doctor wants to inject several ligaments, he will penetrate the skin at two or three points, and then reposition the point of the needle under the skin to reach the ligaments.

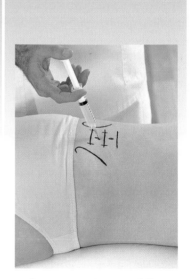

Reference points and lines

The doctor draws reference lines and points on the lower back and then injects the sclerosant into the ligaments (*above*). The horizontal lines are half way between the spinous processes (*left*). The outer vertical lines are over the facet joints.

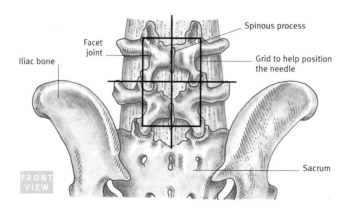

Iliac bone

Facet joint

Spinous process

Grid to help position the needle

Sacrum

FRONT VIEW

local blood flow in the area of the renewed ligaments. Five weeks after the last sclerosant injection the doctor will examine you again and hopefully find you are on the road to recovery.

Results

It takes time for new ligament tissue to grow so do not expect improvement from your back pain until eight weeks after the first injection is given. Some people experience partial relief sooner than this.

The more important question is whether you will be free from back pain in the long term. Some people have excellent results for eight years or more; others do not respond so well. There is no harm in repeating a course of treatment after the benefits of the first course have worn off.

EPIDURAL INJECTIONS

Injections into the epidural space can help disk protrusions causing sciatica and backache that has not responded to rest, pain medication, manipulation, and other physical therapy, including traction, exercise, and massage. If you have severe sciatica and your doctor finds symptoms of a damaged nerve root – numbness of the skin, weakness of certain muscles, and absence of tendon reflex – you may benefit from an epidural. The injection is called an "epidural" because it enters the space between the outer lining of the dura and the bony walls of the spinal canal.

It differs from the epidural given to relieve pain in childbirth in two main ways. Firstly, to treat back pain, most physicians inject the base of the sacrum (childbirth epidurals are given between the lumbar vertebrae). Secondly, they use a weaker solution of local anesthetic and add some steroid. The anesthetic serves to numb the lining of the spinal cord, which is under pressure – usually from a protruding disk or a fragment of disk cartilage. The steroid helps to reduce the inflammation and the bruising of the dural sheath caused by proteins from the ruptured disk. These proteins are enzymes that irritate the dural lining and are toxic to the nerve.

The epidural injection will relieve pain and let you return to normal activities, but it will not help to move the disk protrusion back into place. However, in most cases, the protrusion will wither away gradually by itself, until it stops pressing on the nerve. A minority of people with back pain have a very large disk prolapse, spinal stenosis, or a bone pressing on a nerve. They will not experience lasting benefit from this treatment and, perhaps, will need other approaches.

Procedure

The procedure is simple (*see illustration, p. 104*), and can be performed in the specialist's treatment room. Usually, the injection causes no more than a feeling of pressure in the base of the spine or in the back of the legs, but it may reproduce the sciatic pain at its most severe.

You will be asked to rest for ten minutes on your front followed by ten minutes on your back and the doctor may then test how high your leg can be raised while you hold it straight. After 20 to 30 minutes rest most people can go home (though it is best to have a friend or relative drive you).

If the epidural injection is given via the lower back route (directly between the vertebrae, rather than via the base of the sacrum) a stronger anesthetic is often used that takes longer to wear off and so you may be kept for a few hours before being discharged.

Results

The pain may disappear and never return; it may go for a few hours, return for a few days but fade away by the end of the week; or it may gradually fade over 7 to 14 days. If the injection brings only partial relief after one to two weeks, an alternative route such as nerve blocks may be given.

An epidural that does not work may be due to the disk protrusion pressing too tightly against the nerve root to allow the fluid to pass between the protrusion and the dural membrane, or it may be because the diagnosis was wrong in the first place.

Between 40 and 70 percent of patients obtain some relief. Complications are rare and your condition will not be made worse by reducing the pain in this way. There is a slight risk of absorbing some of the anesthetic fluid, which will cause a temporary numbness and paralysis of the lower legs, but this will clear up in a few hours. Epidural injections do not need to be given under a general anesthetic; in fact, a general anesthetic increases the overall risk of developing complications.

NERVE BLOCKS

An epidural may fail to relieve pain if a nerve is trapped or inflammed in the lateral canal. This can cause pain in your arm or leg without any backache (radiculopathy). An injection of local anesthetic and steroid to the nerve root will block the nerve and reduce inflammation. This technique can also block one or two small nerves that convey pain messages to and from the facet joint and spinal cord.

These injections are very useful for chronic sufferers. They are performed under X-ray control by pain physicians who have a special interest in relieving pain from spinal disorders. If your own doctor cannot help, he may be able to refer you to someone who can.

Procedure

The injection can be given in a treatment room or in an out-patient department. There is no need for a general anesthetic. You will lie on your front on a couch while the physician injects a small amount of local anesthetic together with corticosteroid

Epidural injection

The doctor identifies the base of the sacrum before injecting the anesthetic and steroid mixture into the spinal canal.

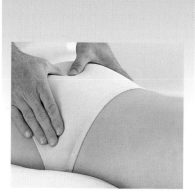

Placing the needle

The buttocks are pulled gently apart to help place the needle correctly (*above*). The mixture reaches the level of the third lumbar vertebra or higher, depending on the volume (*right*).

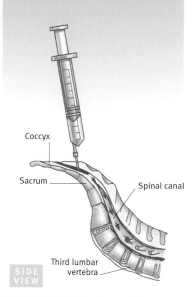

Coccyx

Sacrum

Spinal canal

Third lumbar vertebra

SIDE VIEW

(*see right*). The treatment is not painful, and takes about 20 to 30 minutes.

The only risk is that, very occasionally, the doctor may pierce the dural membrane. He will know at once if he has gone too far and withdraw the needle. Although it will not be painful, you will have to lie flat for 24 hours if this happens, in order to avoid a headache or dizziness caused by an excessive leak of the cerebrospinal fluid.

This is by no means as serious as it may sound. Because of this small risk, it is best to arrange for someone to drive you home. Most specialists perform these nerve blocks using real-time X-rays to guide them, which greatly reduces the risk of puncturing the dural membrane.

Results

If the relevant nerve root has been successfully located, the anesthetic and steroid will provide good pain relief. Sometimes, prolonged or even permanent relief may be obtained. Once again, the results are variable and it is difficult for doctors to predict how well a particular individual will respond. There are no side effects from this nerve block injection since small doses are used and targeted accurately.

FACET JOINT INJECTIONS

Most backaches related to facet joints can be treated successfully with a combination of exercise and improved posture. However, if your symptoms are very severe, you may need an injection. In this case, your doctor will inject a mixture of steroid and local anesthetic into the affected facet joints. The treatment is given in the specialist's office, usually under X-ray control, and you may find it slightly painful.

Unfortunately, if you have osteoarthritis these facet joint injections do not usually provide relief

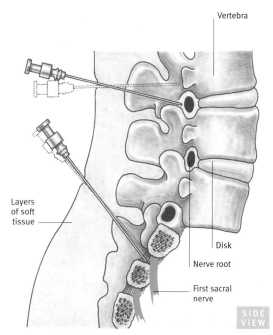

Nerve block
The tip of the needle is positioned in the foramen, where a nerve emerges from the spinal canal, or at the level of the first sacral nerve. The mixture bathes the nerve root to relieve pain and reduce inflammation.

for more than a few months. If you are suffering from this degenerative disease, you may find that one of the newer techniques offered by some pain specialists can bring you more relief.

Radiofrequency facet denervation

In this procedure, the nerve that leads to the joint is anesthetized by a needle, guided under X-ray control. An electrode containing a heat sensor is passed through the needle. This applies a current which heats the nerve just enough to destroy the pain fibers. Several nerve points need to be treated in this way, during a session lasting 30 to 60 minutes. There is some soreness lasting a few days and then lasting pain relief.

Drugs for back pain

Type of drug	Action	Example
Simple pain medication	for relief of mild to moderate pain, act locally and centrally (via the brain)	aspirin, codeine, acetaminophen
Combination drugs	for relief of mild to moderate pain	aspirin, codeine or acetaminophen, combined with cyclobenzaprine
Stronger pain medication	for relief of moderate to severe pain	dihydrocodeine tartrate
Strong nonnarcotic opioids	for relief of severe pain	tramadol
Narcotic analgesics	for relief of severe pain (act via the brain)	morphine or codeine
Muscle relaxants	provide relief by central (brain) sedation and peripheral (muscular) relaxation	diazepam, methocarbamol, cyclobenzaprine
Nonsteroidal anti-inflammatory drugs	reduce pain by inhibiting enzymes at the site of injury or inflammation	ibuprofen, naproxen, diclofenac, etoricoxib, celecoxib
Chemonucleolytics	break down protein and collagen, causing disk to shrink	chymopapain
Steroids (cortisone-type agents)	suppress inflammation	triamcinolone acetonide, triamcinolone hexacetonide, hydrocortisone, methylprednisolone
Low dose tricyclics	counteract nerve pain, muscle tension, poor sleep	amitryptyline, dothiepin
Anticonvulsants	counteract chronic nerve pain	carbamazepine, gabapentin

CHEMONUCLEOLYSIS

This is a treatment for sciatica that is related to disk problems. Chemonucleolysis literally means the chemical breakdown of the nucleus of the disk. It is practiced by relatively few orthopedic surgeons, the majority preferring surgery.

When a minute amount of chymopapain, a protein-digesting enzyme from the papaya fruit, is injected into the center of the disk, the material in the disk starts to break down, so relieving the pressure in the protruded pulp. Within a few weeks, the disk shrinks and the sciatica is relieved.

Procedure

The injection is given in the operating room or radiology department under X-ray control. You do not need a general anesthetic, but a sedative injection may help you relax. The specialist identifies which disk needs treatment with an MRI scan (*see p. 78*) and then injects the chymopapain as you lie either on your front or your side. Soon after, you may experience quite severe pain, and for the first few days you might need pain medication.

Results

Between 50 and 80 percent of patients benefit, but there can be neurological complications or a severe allergic reaction, so if you are allergic to meat tenderizer, melon, or papaya, you cannot receive this treatment.

Recent studies in Europe and Britain show that the risk of complications has been reduced and is less than in surgery. Once a disk has been injected and shrunken, the physical effect is permanent. If, however, the treatment fails to relieve the pain caused by pressure on the nerve root, then surgery will probably be recommended.

Surgery

Surgery to the spine has a very high success rate regardless of the patient's age, due to increasingly accurate diagnosis as much as to improved surgical techniques. The risks from spinal operations are similar to those accompanying all forms of surgery but they are extremely rare.

There is a slim chance of damage to the spinal nerves. Approximately one in 5,000 operations results in nerve damage leading to paralysis. About one in 50 patients suffer from mild yet temporary complications, such as bladder infections. The mortality rate is low, about 0.3 percent, and is usually caused by severe damage to the spinal cord or to a blood clot lodged in the lungs.

Most sciatica patients remain free from root pain ten years after surgery; only 5 to 15 percent need further surgery. Most patients benefit, but the backache is not cured completely so it is important to have realistic expectations.

Operable conditions

The most common spinal operations are those to relieve sciatica. Conditions which may be treated surgically include disk prolapse (usually if it causes sciatica), central or lateral canal stenosis, severe lower back instability, severe facet joint disease, and severe spondylolisthesis. You will probably be offered surgery only after other treatment has failed.

In some circumstances it is best to operate immediately to avoid damage to the spinal cord. These include the following conditions:

• When a large disk prolapse causes pressure on the spinal cord. This would give you severe back pain, severe sciatic pain in one or both legs, marked loss of sensation, and weak muscles in the lower limbs, and bladder and bowel weakness or incontinence. This condition is rare but happens when most of the central, pulpy part of the disk bulges into the spinal canal.

• Occasionally this kind of prolapsed disk may cause only deep pain in the region of the sacrum or coccyx, pain in the crotch and groin areas, and some symptoms of bladder weakness or incontinence. You may not experience leg pain, muscle weakness, and loss of sensation. If your symptoms do not disappear quickly with rest, you may need an MRI scan and surgery.

• Back and/or leg pain of some weeks' duration may, after a while, cause progressive signs of damage to the nerves. If your doctor or specialist examines you regularly to check the degree of muscle weakness and loss of sensation, this should not be missed.

• Sometimes tumors of the vertebrae or infections in the disk space and around the spinal column can produce similar symptoms. These would need urgent surgery or antibiotics.

DISKECTOMY

This operation is used in cases of disk prolapse when the protrusion does not resolve. In a diskectomy, most of the disk is left in place, while the protruding piece is removed. Your doctor may refer you to a specialist who will assess your condition, probably with an MRI or a CT scan. If he is at all uncertain about the diagnosis, the surgeon will not perform the operation.

Procedure

The surgeon removes the protruding part of the disk and any loose fragments and then checks the width of the lateral canal to ensure the nerve root it contains is under no pressure. If the canal is too narrow, he may remove tiny fragments of bone to widen it (*see Decompression, p. 109*). Some surgeons perform this operation through a very small incision not much more than 1in (2cm) long, with the aid of a binocular microscope.

Recuperation

You will be surprised at the dramatic pain relief in your leg if this operation succeeds. The pain from the operative wound is often mild in contrast to the sciatic pain which you have been experiencing over the previous weeks. Within a day the nurses will encourage you to stand up and walk around, but avoid sitting or bending for the first week, since this may stretch the wound.

To prevent scar tissue from forming around the nerve root, you may be advised to practice straight leg lifts (*see p. 133*) several times every day. However, recent studies have cast doubt on this approach to mobilization.

After a week of moving around, your stitches or sutures will be removed. Avoid heavy lifting or

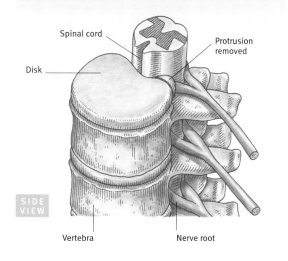

Diskectomy

The main body of the disk is left untouched, but the surgeon removes the part that is protruding and causing pain.

Spinal cord

Protrusion removed

Disk

SIDE VIEW

Vertebra

Nerve root

carrying; if recommended, wear a light lumbar corset to support your back for the first few weeks. Most people can return to light duties or sedentary work within about a month.

Avoid heavy manual work for at least three months. Some specialists would advise against it forever, but if you are young and previously fit, and if you lift and handle things properly, you should be able to manage. Diskectomy causes remarkably little upset to the system in general and people readily return to a normal life.

A disk generally does not become herniated or prolapsed unless it is weakened by recurrent injury. This implies that you should make changes to your lifestyle: avoid becoming overweight, get daily exercises, and follow the advice in Chapter 8.

Most people obtain complete relief from pain in the leg but between a quarter to one half of them still experience some backache. This may be due to minor instability in the lower back which existed before the prolapse, pain from within the damaged disk, and other mechanical disturbances.

DECOMPRESSION

If your spinal canal is too narrow at one point (central or lateral canal stenosis), it might need widening to relieve pressure on nerves. A disk protruding into it can be cured by a diskectomy. However, decompression is needed if you were born with the condition, if bony spurs are growing on the vertebrae, or sometimes when a vertebra shifts and presses on nerves in the central canal, as in spondylolisthesis (see p. 52).

In each case, small pieces of bone are chipped away to leave enough room for the nerves. These conditions can be diagnosed by specialized X-rays and scans, but sometimes a surgeon discovers the problem only during a diskectomy while routinely checking the width of the lateral canal.

Decompression

Two main types of decompression operation remove tiny chips of bone and reduce pressure on the nerves. A laminectomy removes bone from the lamina. A facetectomy removes part of the inner edge of the facet joint.

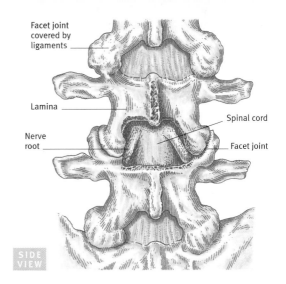

Facet joint covered by ligaments

Lamina

Nerve root

Spinal cord

Facet joint

SIDE VIEW

Procedure

The surgeon exposes the bone and removes tiny amounts of bone from the vertebra. If your spinal canal is too narrow at more than one level, this operation can be extended either up or down without making any other incision. The surgeon may check if the blood circulation to your dural sheath is impaired due to pressure within the spinal canal. If it is, he will extend the operation upward to restore circulation.

Recuperation

You will be able to walk within a day of the operation. After five days you will be allowed home, but will be instructed to avoid strenuous exercise and lifting for about three months.

SPINAL FUSION

If diskography and MRI scans reveal a painful degenerative disk, and you have not responded to comprehensive rehabilitation attempts, you may need a spinal fusion operation.

The goal of spinal fusion is to remove painful disk tissue, which can become so sensitive that almost any movement or pressure hurts, and to stop all movement of the affected segment. But since it leaves a section of the back rigid, doctors are reluctant to consider the operation unless other treatments are unsuccessful.

A fusion operation may also be recommended if you have severe facet joint disease. This often happens when the spine degenerates with age, or when a serious disk prolapse puts extra strain on the facet joints. Spondylolisthesis can be treated with spinal fusion, regardless of whether the back problem is caused by a bone defect or by degenerative change.

Fusion operation

There are two main methods of fusion, with many variations on each one. They involve taking small pieces of bone from some other part of the body (normally the pelvis), and using them as a graft between two vertebrae. Sometimes several segments of the lower back are unstable and are fused by one of these techniques. The spine is usually approached from the back, but increasingly it is reached through an incision in the side or the front of the abdomen.

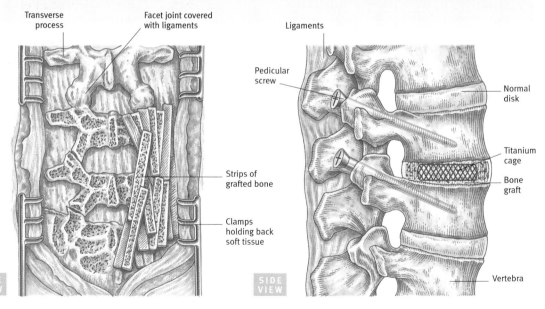

Posterolateral fusion (for posterior column pain)
Strips of bone are placed over the facet joints, between the transverse processes, either on just one side of the vertebra, or on both sides.

Posterior interbody fusion (for anterior column pain)
The entire disk is removed and bits of bone or titanium cages are put in the disk space between the vertebrae to fuse the two vertebrae together.

Insertion of a Harrington rod

An incision is made to expose the entire length of the curve. The spinous processes are removed, and the outer layers of bone are chipped back to leave flaps. A Harrington rod is inserted on the concave side of the curve to straighten it out. Chips of bone are laid all down the curved section, and the flaps of bone are turned down over them.

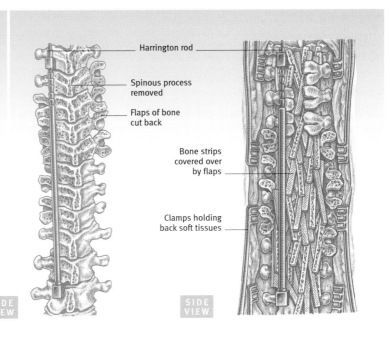

Harrington rod

Spinous process removed

Flaps of bone cut back

Bone strips covered over by flaps

Clamps holding back soft tissues

SIDE VIEW

SIDE VIEW

The operation will probably be recommended to adolescents with severe spondylolisthesis that is damaging their nerves, and causing pain, tingling, or numbness in their legs. Adults suffering from degenerative spondylolisthesis may also need a fusion operation. However, if the only symptom is leg pain, without any accompanying back pain, you could be treated with decompression.

Recuperation

Spinal fusion is more traumatic than a diskectomy. You will need to mobilize more gradually over the ensuing weeks. If instrumentation (screws) is not used, you may have to use a rigid back brace for six to eight weeks. The aim of this aftercare is to let the fusion become solid. It takes anything from six months to a year to achieve the full effects, so you should not look for immediate relief of symptoms.

In the past, the operation was often performed at the same time as a standard diskectomy to treat a prolapsed disk, in order to prevent further disk herniation or backache. It is now recognized that this combination is no more successful than simply removing the prolapse.

Some surgeons choose a fusion operation if, following back surgery such as decompression or diskectomy, the patient still complains of severe and incapacitating low back pain.

SURGERY FOR SCOLIOSIS

In most cases of scoliosis (see p. 52), the curve is very slight, and may cause no pain at all. However, in very severe cases structural scoliosis can produce considerable deformity, and you may need surgery to straighten your spine. The operation is most commonly done in early adolescence, since this is when the most severe spinal curvatures develop.

Procedure

The most common form of surgical treatment for scoliosis is the insertion of a Harrington rod (see above). This telescopic metal rod is wedged alongside the vertebrae on the concave side of the curve. During the operation, the rod is elongated to open the curve, and then the entire curved section is fused with chips of bone taken from the hip bone. If the scoliosis is very severe, you may need a compression Harrington rod on the other side of the curve.

In another method, the spine is approached from the front, and the disks between the vertebrae forming the curve are removed. Bolts are drilled transversely through the vertebrae and then crimped onto a steel cable lying down the convex side. The whole assembly is then tightened, thus pulling the spine straight.

Recuperation

If you have either of these operations, you will be in the hospital for several days, and off from school or work for a month. You will have to avoid sports for between six months and a year.

The operations will result in a very stiff back. In most cases, they will leave the ribs slightly prominent on one side. If this is particularly deforming, you can have cosmetic surgery to reduce the prominence.

SURGERY FOR COCCYDYNIA

If pain resulting from a fall on the coccyx has not cleared up after several months, surgery is sometimes necessary. This involves removing the last two or three segments of the coccyx. If there has been a fracture, it is possible that it has not reunited and the loose fragment can be removed, giving relief from pain.

Recuperation

The operation is relatively minor and you can be up and walking about in a few days. Obviously, you will not be able to sit up until the wound from

the operation has healed, but you can expect to be back at work in most occupations within two to three weeks.

SURGERY OF THE NECK

The problems that occur in the neck are much the same as those in the lower spine. Doctors are more reluctant to recommend surgery, though, since any damage to the spinal cord in the neck could be fatal or result in the paralysis of all four limbs.

However, in some conditions, there is a risk of the spinal cord becoming damaged through compression of the nerves, so you might need an urgent operation. These conditions include a disk protruding into the central spinal canal, dislodged bones, or bony spurs (osteophytes) pressing on nerves, or a tumor.

Fusion operation

If a disk prolapse in your neck does not recover after some months, you may need surgery. Nerves in the neck can be compressed by spurs growing on the vertebrae (cervical spondylosis). This may damage your spinal cord, particularly if segments in your neck are too mobile.

The degree of mobility in your neck can be assessed by a specialized X-ray to find out whether a fusion operation could improve your condition. You will also have an MRI scan to determine the width of the spinal canal.

This operation will probably be done by an orthopedic or neurosurgeon who will remove the disk through an incision in the front of the neck. This surgery is usually performed under a microscope.

Because disks in the neck are much smaller than those in the lower back, a much smaller space is left between the vertebrae once the disk is removed. The bones fuse naturally after this operation, and a bone graft is unnecessary.

A fusion operation on the neck has a very high success rate. Almost 100 percent of patients with a cervical disk prolapse are relieved of pain, and about 90 percent of those with lateral canal stenosis (*see p. 57*) benefit.

You will need to stay in hospital for only three or four days, but you will have to wear a rigid collar for about two months. If you have a sedentary job, you should be able to return to work within a week or two, but you should not return to work which involves heavy lifting and carrying for two months or so, to allow the vertebrae to fuse completely.

Fracture dislocation

A vertebra in the neck can sometimes become displaced after a fracture. If it does not slip back into place immediately, you will need traction to the skull to prevent damage to your spinal cord. Once the displacement has reduced, an operation will be performed either to fuse the damaged segments with bone grafts, or to fix them with wire. You will need to wear a neck brace for at least three months.

FAILURE OF SURGERY

If there is no improvement in your back problem immediately after your operation, there are several possible reasons why:

● The wrong diagnosis was made. This is unlikely if the specialist operated on the clinical picture confirmed by a scan, and not simply on the basis of abnormalities shown on scans.

● The symptoms are mainly psychological, or you have developed a chronic pain disorder.

● The operation was performed at the wrong level.

● In an operation for a disk prolapse, a second prolapsed disk may be present, or a fragment of the disk may remain in the lateral canal.

If relief was temporary, but your symptoms return, there are several possible explanations:

● The area operated on may have become infected.

● A cyst may have developed on the lining of the spinal cord.

● You may have developed arachnoiditis or scar tissue around the nerve.

● You might have lateral canal stenosis (*see p. 57*).

● The area that was operated on may have become unstable, causing facet joint pain.

● If the operation was to treat a prolapsed disk, a second disk prolapse at the same level may have developed.

● In a spinal fusion operation, the most likely explanation is that the surgeon has stabilized only the posterior column when you have anterior pain. Alternatively, the bones may not have fused solidly, a false joint may have developed between two segments of bone graft, or there could be a prolapsed disk above the fused level.

These problems occur in only five to ten percent of patients who have surgery, but for some conditions the success rate is lower. About 20 percent of fusion operations for spondylolisthesis result in the formation of a false joint. If spinal surgery fails to relieve your symptoms, the advice on coping with pain may be useful (*see Chapter 9*).

Expectations

To reiterate, do not expect total and permanent relief from pain after an operation, or you are likely to be disappointed. If the operation is successful, and most are, the pain should certainly be dramatically reduced, and you should have much better mobility. To reap the greatest benefit, however, you must follow any advice given by the surgeon or the physical therapist on how to take care of your back, and you should use the self-help measures described in Chapters 8 and 9.

7

Exercises

Exercising your back is important for recovering from an acute backache, and may help those with chronic back pain. Some exercises in this chapter are designed to help with specific back problems while others are for general back care.

The chart on page 116 will help you decide which exercises are most appropriate for your condition. Start with the more gentle ones but stop immediately if your back pain increases. If you are unsure whether you are doing an exercise correctly, ask a professional to

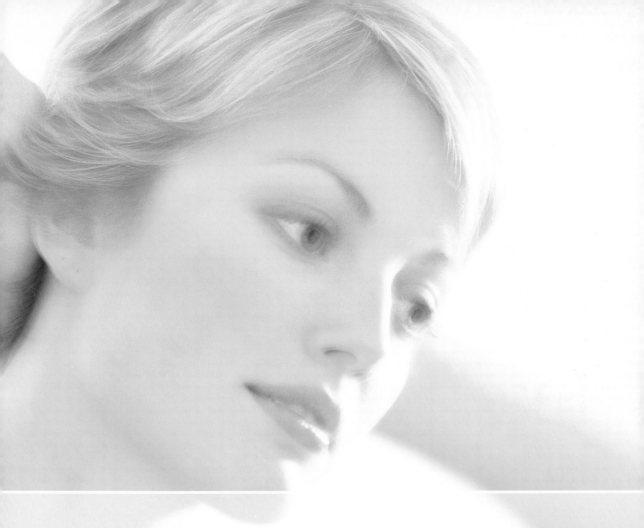

watch you. After an acute attack, begin exercising as soon as you can move without undue pain. You may ache and feel slightly stiff but don't let this stop you. If you can, practice the exercises two or three times a day, but in general practice a few at least once a day. The number of recommended repetitions is what an average person should be able to manage. Don't worry if you can manage only two or three repetitions to start with. As you become more fit, try to repeat the exercises 20 or even 30 times per session.

Choosing the right exercise

If you are suffering from an episode of acute back pain, start with the appropriate exercises in the left hand column as soon as you can move without too much pain – probably about a day after the attack began. Progress to the exercises in the middle column when the severe pain has subsided. The exercises in the third column are for stretching and strengthening, to help you to avoid back trouble.

Condition	During acute attack	After severe pain	Prevention
Acute lumbar pain (caused by disk syndrome)	Pelvic tilt Passive extension* Mountain and sag	Passive extension* Standing extension Low back stretch* Side gliding Gentle rotation Side bending	Hamstring stretches Abdominal exercises Leg exercises
Acute torticollis (caused by disk or facet joint)	Passive extension*	Retraction and lengthening Passive extension	
Acute pain in the leg	Pelvic tilt Passive extension*	Passive extension* Low back stretch* Gentle twisting	Hamstring stretches Abdominal exercises Leg exercises
Lumbar instability	Pelvic tilt	Passive extension Low back stretch Stabilizing exercises	Abdominal exercises Leg exercises Back strengthening
Facet joint disease	Pelvic tilt	Low back stretch	Abdominal exercises Standing pelvic tilt
Strained muscles		Gentle rotation Side bending Low back stretch	
Tense muscles	Low back stretch Gentle rotation Side bending Leg muscle stretches Neck stretches		
Trigger points	Specific exercises to stretch the affected muscles		

*If your pain increases after six repetitions, do not continue the exercise. If pain persists, seek medical attention.

Therapeutic exercises for lower backs

These may help acute pain in the lower back or sciatica. Always follow your physical therapist's or doctor's advice about exercising your back. But if you have recurrent attacks and are familiar with the exercises, or if you feel that your attack is not sufficiently severe to warrant a consultation, then it may be worth trying any of the following exercises. Begin the exercises about a day after the pain first started, but stop immediately if the pain increases or spreads away from your spine.

Pelvic tilt

This helps most types of acute lumbar pain by relieving pressure on the facet joints and gently stretching the muscles and ligaments of the back. It strengthens the abdominal muscles that indirectly support the spine. If practiced regularly, it encourages better posture. Do it on the floor at first, but later try it standing up. If it's easier, support your legs on cushions in the Fowler position (see p. 66).

1 Lie on the floor with your arms at your sides, your feet flat on the floor and your legs bent at a comfortable angle.

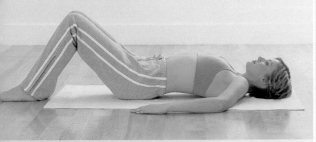

2 Gently press the small of your back against the floor and tilt your pubic bone upward by tightening your abdominal and pelvic floor muscles. Hold for at least six seconds, then relax slowly. Repeat up to ten times.

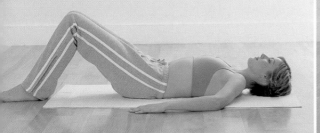

Passive extension

This helps many kinds of backache brought on by sitting. Don't try it if it increases your pain. If bending backward or staying upright is difficult because you are already stuck in a stooped position, lower yourself slowly until you are lying face down and relax for a few minutes before you start. Try the exercise two or three times initially.

1 Lie face down with your hands flat on the floor and level with your shoulders as if you were about to do a push-up.

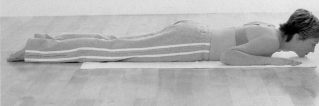

2 Push up with your arms, leaving your hips on the floor. Lift your head and shoulders as high as you can. Let your back sag in. Breathe out, then slowly lower your trunk, using your arm muscles only. Repeat up to ten times.

Let your spine arch progressively more with each repetition

Side gliding

This was developed by physical therapist Robin Mackenzie to help people with acute lumbago whose pelvis tilts or lists to one side. Look in a mirror: if your right hip is more prominent, this exercise should help you pull your pelvis to the left and glide your trunk to the right. If your left hip is more prominent, do the exercise the other way around.

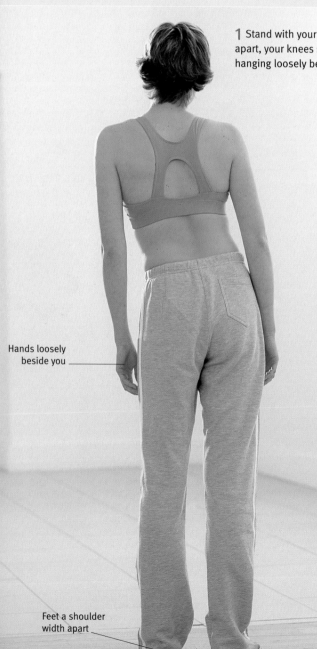

1 Stand with your feet shoulder width apart, your knees straight, and your hands hanging loosely beside you.

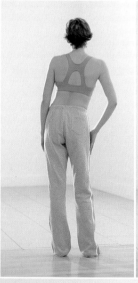

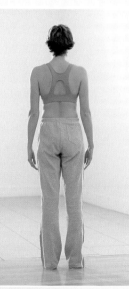

Hands loosely beside you

Feet a shoulder width apart

2 Slowly bring your hips across to the left. Move your shoulders (keep them horizontal) to the right. This may be painful and cause twinges, and the muscles will tighten up in resistance. Stop if the pain increases in the back or legs. Maintain steady, relaxed breathing and sustain the stretch.

3 Relax and stand up straight. Don't let your hips slip back to the right again. Repeat ten times, until you can return to a neutral position with no tilt. Now perform a series of standing extension movements (*see far right*).

Low back stretch

This helps if you have strained a facet joint and the surrounding muscles are tight and aching. But avoid it if your pain is caused by a disk protrusion.

1 Lie down and do a basic pelvic tilt (*see p. 117*). Then draw your knees up toward your chest, keeping your lower back flat.

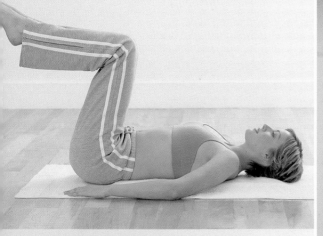

2 Grasp your legs and squeeze your knees to your chest. Breathe deeply. Maintain the squeeze for at least seven seconds. Release the legs, lowering them slowly. Keep the knees bent and your back firmly pressed to the floor. If you feel a painful twinge, try lowering one leg at a time.

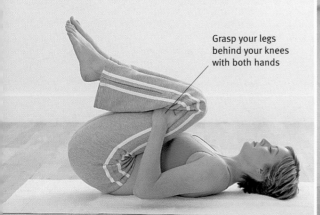

Grasp your legs behind your knees with both hands

Standing extension

This gently arches your lower back, and should be performed every couple of hours throughout the day. Stop if it increases the pain. Try the passive extension exercise (*see p. 117*) instead.

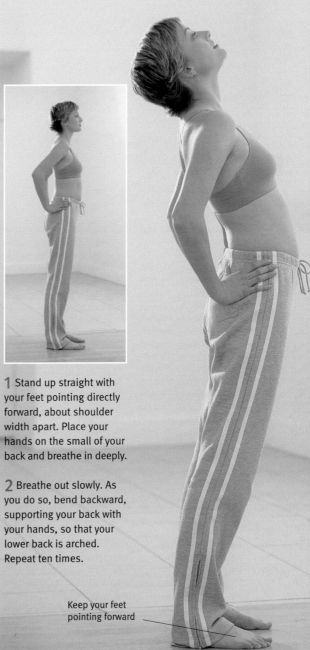

1 Stand up straight with your feet pointing directly forward, about shoulder width apart. Place your hands on the small of your back and breathe in deeply.

2 Breathe out slowly. As you do so, bend backward, supporting your back with your hands, so that your lower back is arched. Repeat ten times.

Keep your feet pointing forward

Mobilizing exercises

These exercises are generally useful for improving and maintaining mobility, which is essential to a healthy back. They can be helpful in most back conditions. Stop immediately if an exercise increases your pain. The mountain and sag exercise below, and the rotation and bending exercises on page 122, gently stretch your muscles and prevent your spinal joints from becoming stiff.

Mountain and sag

This rhythmic exercise of the lower back helps in most cases of acute lower back pain, caused by either facet joint or disk problems. If the extreme sag position is painful, let your spine drop to a point just before you know you are going to feel the twinge.

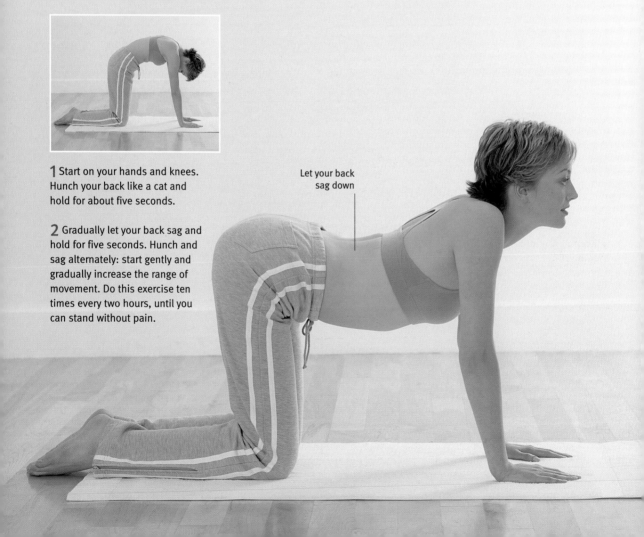

1 Start on your hands and knees. Hunch your back like a cat and hold for about five seconds.

2 Gradually let your back sag and hold for five seconds. Hunch and sag alternately: start gently and gradually increase the range of movement. Do this exercise ten times every two hours, until you can stand without pain.

Let your back sag down

Gentle rotation

This improves general mobility and is particularly useful for relaxing the muscles around the back and pelvic areas. It also relieves facet joint pain by stretching the capsules and ligaments around the facet joints in the lower back: those on the left will be stretched as you drop your knees to the right, and vice versa.

1 Lie on your back with your knees bent, your feet flat on the floor, and your arms by your sides, as for the pelvic tilt (*see p. 117*). Press your lower back against the floor.

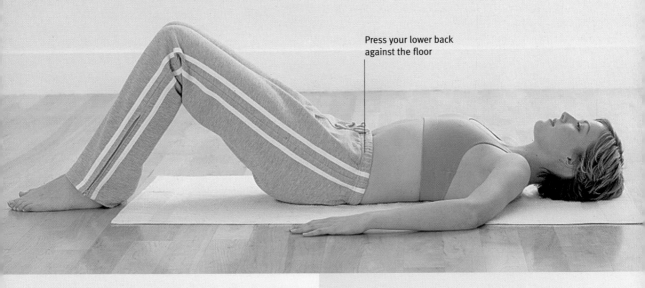

Press your lower back against the floor

2 Keeping your knees together, lift them until they are above your navel.

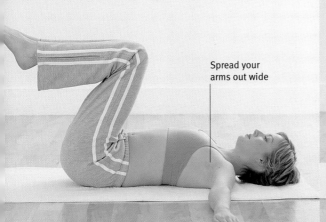

Spread your arms out wide

3 Let your legs flop slowly over to the right as far as they will go. Breathe slowly and deeply. Let the legs drop a little further with each breath. Hold for a minute. Bring your legs back up and lower them to the other side. Repeat the exercise, twisting to each side ten times.

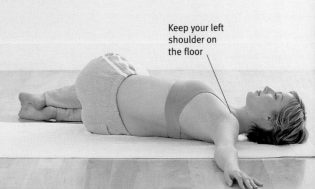

Keep your left shoulder on the floor

Trunk rotation

Rotating the trunk of your body to each side will gently stretch your spinal muscles. Turn to the right, then to the left. Repeat the exercise five times.

1 Sit astride a chair, straighten your spine, cross your arms, and breathe in deeply.

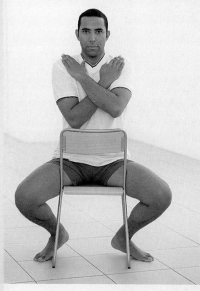

2 As you breathe out, slowly turn to the right as far as you can.

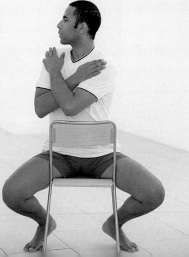

Side bending

This exercise mobilizes the whole spine. The bending movements stretch the muscles around the waist and side of the trunk.

1 Stand with your feet shoulder width apart, your knees slightly bent, and your arms by your sides.

Keep the upper arm as close as you can to the side of your head

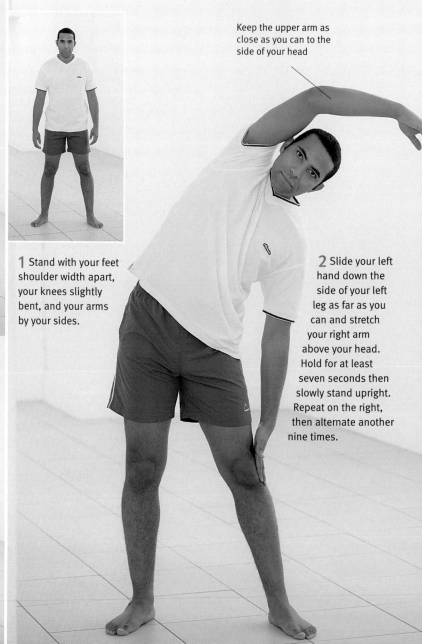

2 Slide your left hand down the side of your left leg as far as you can and stretch your right arm above your head. Hold for at least seven seconds then slowly stand upright. Repeat on the right, then alternate another nine times.

The lumbar pelvic rhythm

This stretching exercise is more strenuous than the previous mobilizing exercises, so don't try it until your acute back pain is on the mend. The goal is to master the rhythm. When you bend your back, your upper back should bend first, then the lower back, and finally the pelvis and hips. You should straighten up in reverse order. Bending in this reverse order puts controlled strain on the lower back, because half of the body passes well in front of the center of gravity.

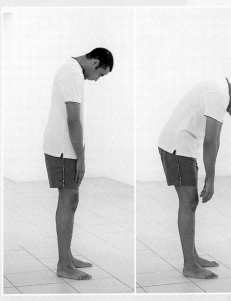

1 Stand with your feet together. Bend your neck until your chin touches your chest.

2 Slowly slide your hands down the front of your legs – curling your back segment by segment – as far as they will naturally go.

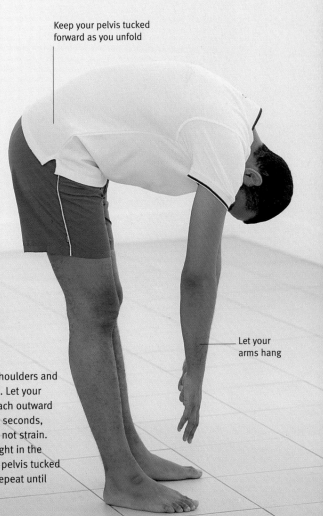

Keep your pelvis tucked forward as you unfold

Let your arms hang

3 Relax your neck and shoulders and keep your knees straight. Let your muscles go loose with each outward breath. Hang for 10 to 15 seconds, stretching out gently. Do not strain. Uncurl slowly to the upright in the reverse order. Keep your pelvis tucked forward as you unfold. Repeat until you master the rhythm.

Abdominal exercises

These exercises strengthen particular groups of abdominal muscles. The pelvic tilt (*see p. 117*) and oblique abdominal exercise are isometric (iso = same; meter = length), so called because a maximum concentration of muscle power is combined with a minimum change in length. During the exercises you hold certain muscles rigid while hardly moving that part of your body.

Oblique abdominal exercise

This is good for sports such as golf, which require turning movements of the trunk. It is generally helpful for all back conditions, since it tones up the abdominal muscles. It is also useful for trimming weight from the sides of the abdomen and improving the waistline.

1 Lie down with your legs bent and press your lower back against the floor, as for the pelvic tilt (*see p. 117*).

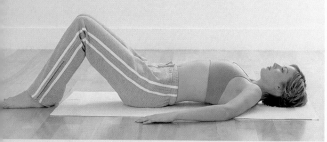

2 Raise your left knee to the vertical. Rest your right hand on the knee. Keep your lower back on the floor and push with your arm and resist with your knee. Maintain the tension for at least seven seconds. Relax slowly, lowering your leg to the floor. Repeat with your right leg and left arm. Practice ten times on each side.

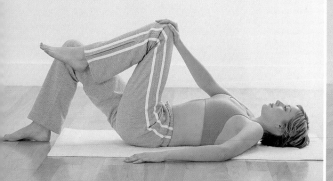

Head and shoulder lift

This benefits all back conditions. It is appropriate for people whose abdominal muscles require more strengthening or for those who wish to trim excess weight from the abdomen. It is less strenuous than a full sit-up, but don't try it while your back is hurting.

1 Lie on your back with your legs bent and press your lower back against the floor, as for the pelvic tilt (*see p. 117*).

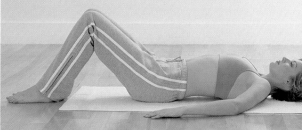

2 Raise your head until your chin touches your chest. Reach forward with your arms toward your lower legs, raising your shoulders as high as you can. Keep your lower back on the floor. Hold the raised position for at least seven seconds. Relax slowly, uncurling the back first, then the shoulders and the neck. Repeat ten times in a session.

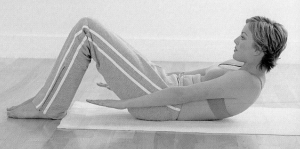

Oblique crunches

These are more dynamic exercises, requiring flexibility, stamina, and mobilization. If you are unsure whether it is appropriate for you, don't attempt it and consult your doctor or physical therapist.

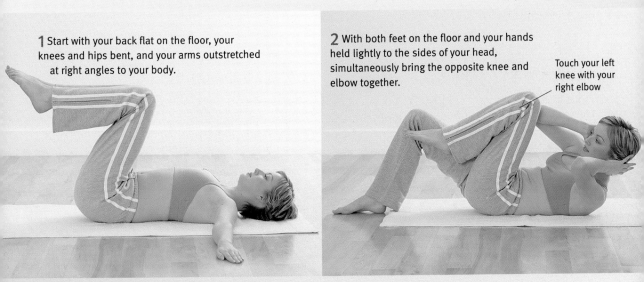

1 Start with your back flat on the floor, your knees and hips bent, and your arms outstretched at right angles to your body.

2 With both feet on the floor and your hands held lightly to the sides of your head, simultaneously bring the opposite knee and elbow together.

Touch your left knee with your right elbow

3 Alternate the movement at a steady pace between 30 and 60 times a minute. Each time make sure you curl up and rotate your trunk and avoid grasping your head or neck. Breathe rhythmically throughout. Follow with gentle rotations of the hips and legs (*see p. 121*).

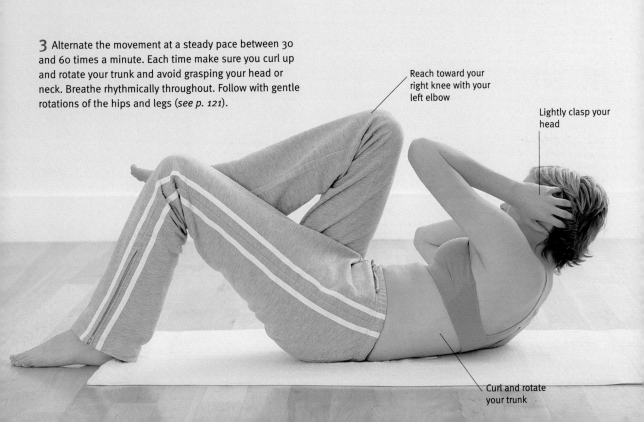

Reach toward your right knee with your left elbow

Lightly clasp your head

Curl and rotate your trunk

Cycling

This exercise involves considerable control of your pelvic position. First perform the pelvic tilt (*see p. 117*), keeping your lower back on the floor at all times. Then move to the first step of oblique crunches (*see p. 125*), with your knees and hips bent at a right angle.

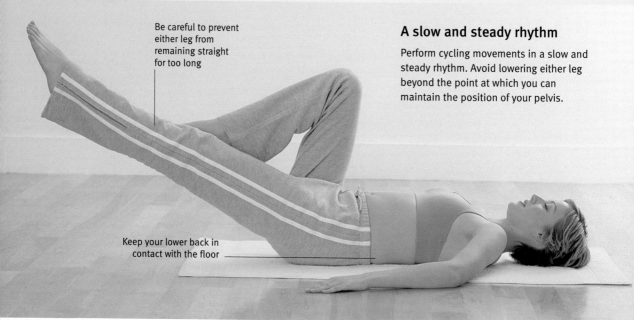

Be careful to prevent either leg from remaining straight for too long

Keep your lower back in contact with the floor

A slow and steady rhythm

Perform cycling movements in a slow and steady rhythm. Avoid lowering either leg beyond the point at which you can maintain the position of your pelvis.

Muscle balance

Postural stabilization is taught by specially trained physical therapists and is related to the Alexander technique and Pilates. The goal is to improve spinal stability by helping you activate the deepest layers of muscles (multifidus, transversus abdominis) which control posture. In acute episodes these muscles weaken and do not automatically recover when the pain goes. The pelvic tilt (*see p. 117*), the all 4's (*see p. 127*), and this Swiss ball exercise are three examples of the kind of exercises used. They are not "hard work" but, like any new skill, they require concentration.

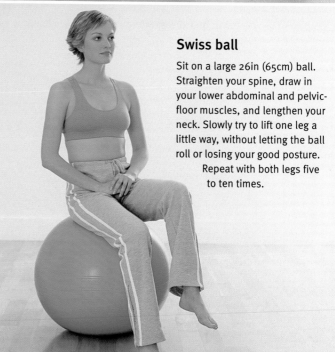

Swiss ball

Sit on a large 26in (65cm) ball. Straighten your spine, draw in your lower abdominal and pelvic-floor muscles, and lengthen your neck. Slowly try to lift one leg a little way, without letting the ball roll or losing your good posture. Repeat with both legs five to ten times.

Back-strengthening exercises

Chronic back pain can lead to weak back muscles. The traditional exercises for strengthening back muscles tend to raise pressure in the disks and facet joints of the lower back. They may aggravate the condition if started too intensively or too soon after an acute flare-up. Evidence suggests that dynamic strengthening of the extensors (muscles used to straighten up the back and limbs) and recruitment of the deep stabilizing muscles can help in preventing a relapse.

All 4's lifting one leg

Core stability comes from learning to use the deep abdominal muscle layer (transversus) to support the lumbar spine while moving the limbs. This exercise helps you to use your buttock muscles more independently.

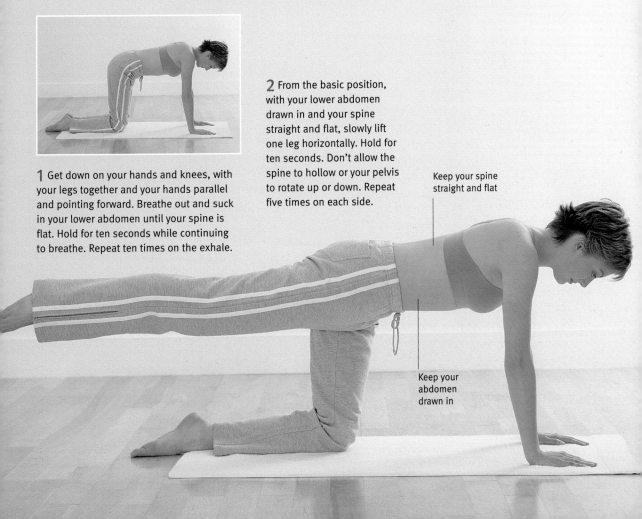

2 From the basic position, with your lower abdomen drawn in and your spine straight and flat, slowly lift one leg horizontally. Hold for ten seconds. Don't allow the spine to hollow or your pelvis to rotate up or down. Repeat five times on each side.

1 Get down on your hands and knees, with your legs together and your hands parallel and pointing forward. Breathe out and suck in your lower abdomen until your spine is flat. Hold for ten seconds while continuing to breathe. Repeat ten times on the exhale.

Keep your spine straight and flat

Keep your abdomen drawn in

Alternate limb lift

This exercise is one of the many exercises which train the back, transversus, and hip girdle muscles to work together to improve stability and posture.

Hold the parallel

From step 2 of the all 4's position, stretch out the opposite arm and leg parallel to the floor. Hold for ten seconds, then lower. Repeat with the other arm and leg. Repeat five times each side.

Keep the spine flat and the pelvis stable

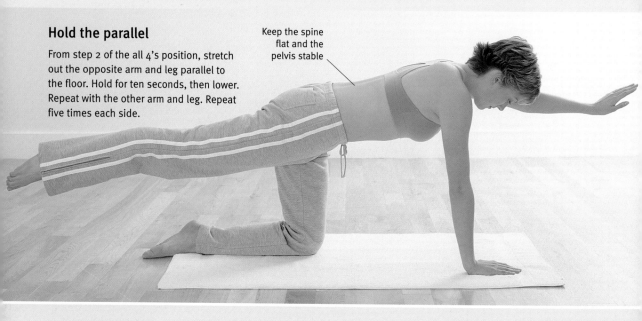

Horizontal lift

In this exercise, do not raise your legs or shoulders above the horizontal, since this would increase the stress on your facet joints.

1 Lie face down on a pillow across a firm table, with someone holding your ankles to keep your legs in place. Lift your whole trunk until your body is horizontal. Do not pass beyond this point.

2 Lower your trunk and relax. Repeat ten times in one session. Increase gradually over three months to 100 repetitions.

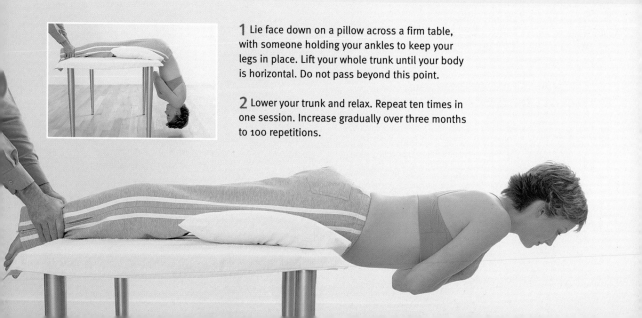

Both legs lift

Like the horizontal lift on the previous page, this exercise is vigorous and makes a good contribution to the long-term prevention of lower back pain.

1 Lie forward over a firm table and hold on to the sides with both hands. Bend your knees so that the weight of your legs is held entirely by your back muscles.

The entire weight of your legs is held by the muscles of your back

Keep your feet together

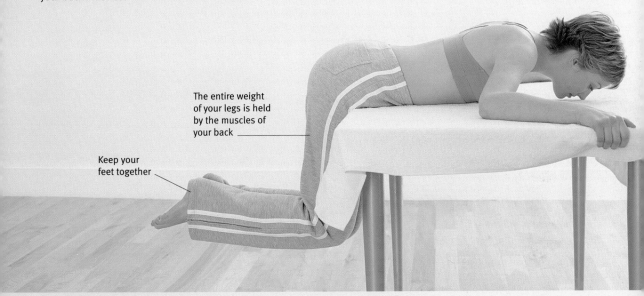

2 Extend your knees and raise your legs outward to a horizontal position and then return. Repeat this ten times during the first session. Subsequently, increase the number of repetitions gradually to between 50 and 100 over a three-month period.

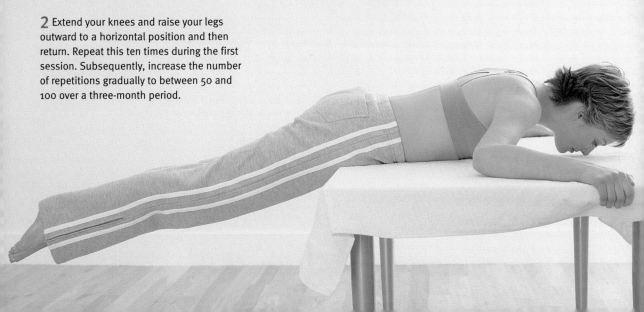

Buttock and leg exercises

Sometimes the mobility of the spine is restricted not just by stiffness in the joints and ligaments, but also because the muscles are not flexible enough. People with chronic low back pain tend to develop tighter hamstring muscles and sometimes even the calf muscles in the lower leg become tighter. In addition, inflexible leg muscles make you prone to back trouble because you will tend to lift and bend in the wrong way, so these exercises, particularly the hamstring stretches, can be used preventatively.

Squats

Don't worry if you can only do two or three repetitions at first. Performing the squats two to three times a day over a few days will increase your strength until you can manage as many as 20 repetitions.

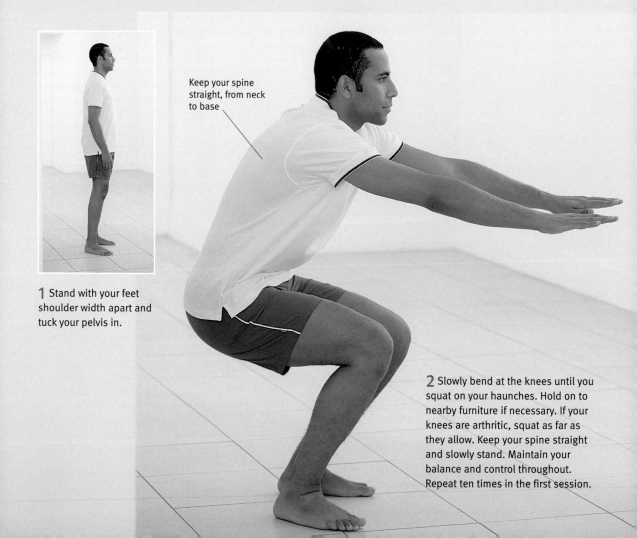

Keep your spine straight, from neck to base

1 Stand with your feet shoulder width apart and tuck your pelvis in.

2 Slowly bend at the knees until you squat on your haunches. Hold on to nearby furniture if necessary. If your knees are arthritic, squat as far as they allow. Keep your spine straight and slowly stand. Maintain your balance and control throughout. Repeat ten times in the first session.

Hip hitch

This simple exercise helps to strengthen the buttock and hip muscles to improve stable transfer of weight from one leg to the other.

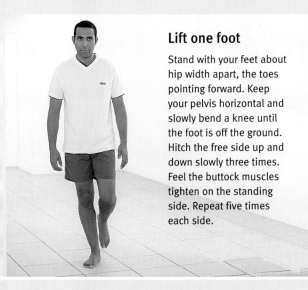

Lift one foot

Stand with your feet about hip width apart, the toes pointing forward. Keep your pelvis horizontal and slowly bend a knee until the foot is off the ground. Hitch the free side up and down slowly three times. Feel the buttock muscles tighten on the standing side. Repeat five times each side.

Calf muscle stretch

This increases the elasticity of the calf muscles and Achilles tendons at the back of the ankles.

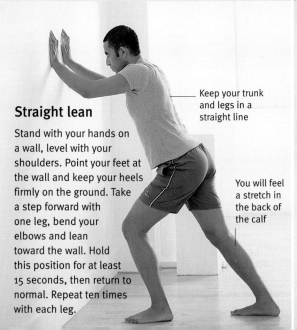

Straight lean

Stand with your hands on a wall, level with your shoulders. Point your feet at the wall and keep your heels firmly on the ground. Take a step forward with one leg, bend your elbows and lean toward the wall. Hold this position for at least 15 seconds, then return to normal. Repeat ten times with each leg.

Keep your trunk and legs in a straight line

You will feel a stretch in the back of the calf

Standing hamstring stretch

This exercise will not strain your lower back. You may find this exercise easier if you hold your leg behind your knee to give it a little extra support.

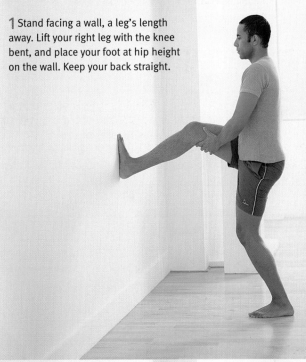

1 Stand facing a wall, a leg's length away. Lift your right leg with the knee bent, and place your foot at hip height on the wall. Keep your back straight.

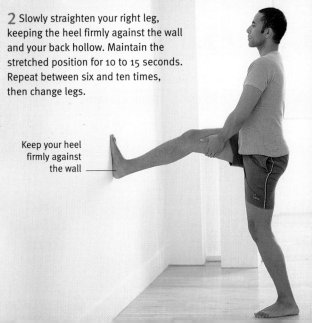

2 Slowly straighten your right leg, keeping the heel firmly against the wall and your back hollow. Maintain the stretched position for 10 to 15 seconds. Repeat between six and ten times, then change legs.

Keep your heel firmly against the wall

Quads stretch

The quadriceps muscles are powerful leg muscles. They are prone to shortening with inactivity as well as vigorous activity and need regular stretching.

Tilt backward

Stand up straight with your back toward a firm table (or couch). Place one foot on the table behind you. Keeping your legs parallel, tilt your pelvis backward and feel the stretch throughout the front of your thigh. Hold this position for 15 seconds. Perform the exercise five times with each foot on the table.

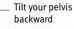
Tilt your pelvis backward

Hip flexor stretch

The psoas muscles (*see p. 18*) shorten with prolonged sitting, creating a muscle imbalance. Stretching them reduces strain on the lower back. Start by sitting on the edge of a firm padded table, with your legs hanging over. Then lie back and rest your head on a pillow.

1 Lift up one leg and bend it at the knee. Grip the thigh and bring the knee close to your chest.

2 Bring the other leg to the horizontal. Hold for 20 seconds. Relax at the hip and knee, letting it drop to achieve a full stretch for 15–20 seconds. Do this five times on each side.

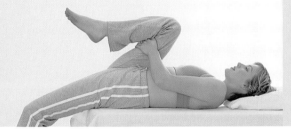

Lying hamstring stretch

Some hamstring stretches tend to pull on the joints of the lower back but this exercise does not. So if your back is at all painful or fragile, start with this exercise.

1 Lie on your back with your arms beside you and your legs straight. Lift your right leg, bending the knee to a right angle.

Keep your thigh vertical

2 Slowly straighten your right leg as much as you can. Hold for 10 to 15 seconds to let the muscle relax and stretch. Lower your leg slowly and repeat with your left leg. Repeat the exercise another nine times on either side.

Keep your left leg firmly on the floor

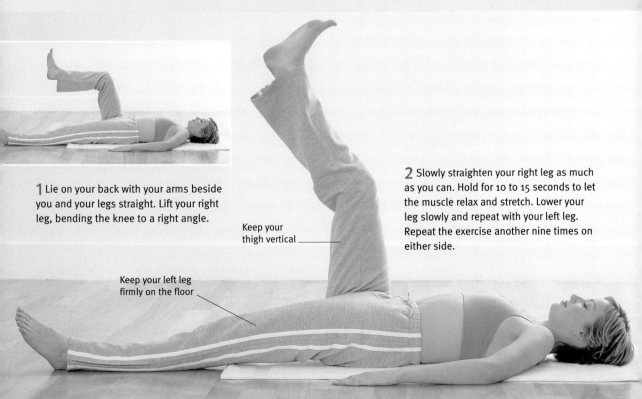

Neck exercises

Several exercises can help if you are prone to neck problems. Sometimes, after poor posture has been sustained for a long time, the muscles will not relax at all and will ache continuously. This can cause severe pain, headaches, tingling, and cold sensations in that area. If this is the case, the following neck exercises may help encourage your muscles to relax. Try to follow them up with a massage (*see pp. 70–71*). The passive extension exercise is more likely to relieve pain caused by disk bulge. The neck retraction and lengthening exercise will help to relax your neck muscles; with regular practice it should encourage you to hold your head correctly.

Passive extension

This allows your head to provide traction for your neck. Do not perform without consulting your doctor. Do not try if you are middle-aged, elderly, and/or are prone to dizzy spells when you turn your head or look up. Do not remove your hands to complete this exercise if your head does not drop all the way back in Step 3.

1 Lie on your back on a firm bed or a flat couch, with your shoulders on the edge, and your head, supported by your hands, projecting over the end.

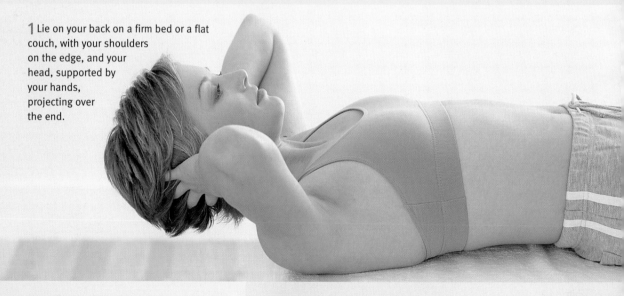

2 Breathe out. Lower your head gently. Let your hands take the weight of your head as you completely relax your neck muscles.

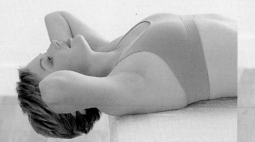

3 If you can lower your head all the way back, your neck will be fully extended and you can remove your hands. Hold the position for about a minute at first. After three or four attempts in a day try holding for longer. To get up, put your hands under your head and gently raise and support your head until your spine is straight. Roll over on to your stomach and stand up.

Retraction and lengthening

This helps to reduce postural pain. If practiced regularly, it may prevent neck strain by encouraging better posture. Try it whenever you catch yourself holding your head forward with your chin jutting out.

Active range of motion

If you have experienced any neck strain or sprain, practice this exercise regularly to help you regain your normal range of motion. Before you start, perform the neck retraction and lengthening exercise (*see left*).

1 Look straight ahead, pull your chin back, and lengthen your neck. Make the crown of your head the highest point and elongate the distance between your shoulders and your ears.

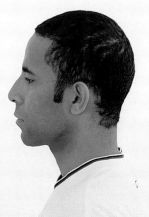

1 Bend your head slowly forward and backward a few times.

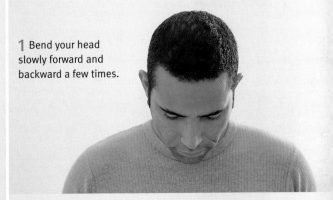

2 Bend your head sideways, trying to bring your ear down to your shoulder. Repeat each side several times.

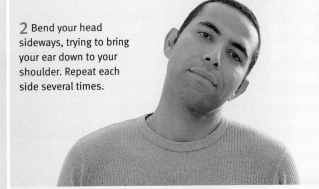

2 Raise your shoulders then lower them slowly while breathing out. Continue until your shoulders feel relaxed, keeping your neck straight and your chin tucked in.

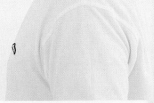
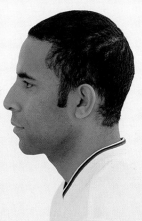
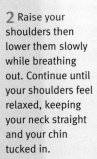

3 Rotate your head slowly to the right, maintaining the retracted and lengthened neck position throughout. Repeat each side several times.

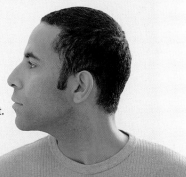

Isometric exercises

These three exercises strengthen your neck muscles by using your hands to prevent your head from moving. Do not do them if your neck muscles are already very tense, since they could make the muscles even more tense. All three can be done either sitting or standing.

Resisted neck extension

Fold your hands behind your head and push your head back as far as possible while resisting with your hands. Hold for six seconds and then relax. Repeat ten times.

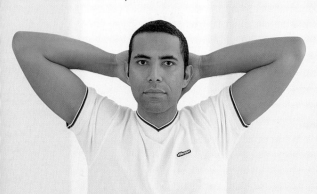

Resisted side bend

Push your head against the heel of your hand while resisting with your arm. Maintain maximum tension for at least six seconds. Repeat ten times on each side.

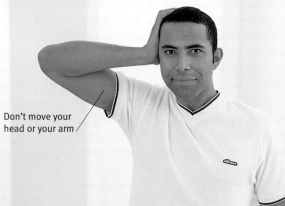

Don't move your head or your arm

Rotation

Place the heel of your right hand over your right temple and the heel of the left hand toward the back of your head on the other side. Try to turn your head toward the right, resisting with both arms. Hold for six seconds Repeat ten times and then repeat the exercise, trying to the left.

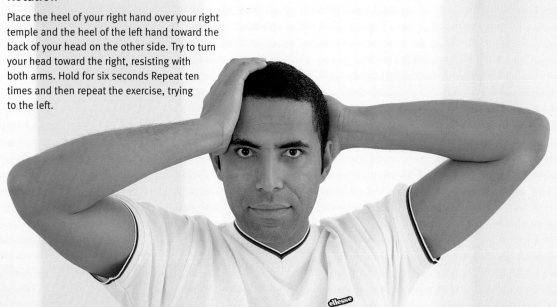

Neck stretch

This exercise uses the weight of your head to stretch your neck muscles; it will reduce tension in your neck and shoulders. The instructions here start with stretching the left side.

1 Sit on an upright chair and hold the seat with your left hand. Keep your left arm straight, and without raising your left shoulder, slowly lean your head and neck as far to the right as you can. Feel the stretch. Hold it for at least 15 seconds and return to the upright position. Repeat several times.

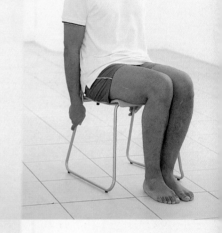

2 Repeat the same sequence on the opposite side, leaning to the left as far as you can.

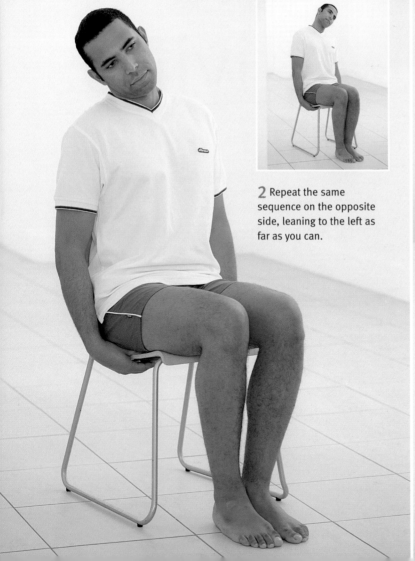

Neck stretch

The key to effective stretching is lengthening the whole spine, lifting the chest, and maintaining a downward pull on the shoulder girdle via a firm hand hold. Repeat these steps on the opposite sides.

1 Hold the back of the chair with both hands and move your head to the left and slightly forward.

2 Hold the front of the chair with both hands and incline your head to the right and slightly backward.

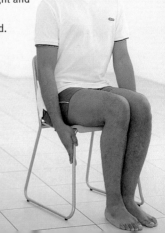

8

Posture and Everyday Activities

A great deal of chronic or recurring back pain is due to poor posture. In a way this is heartening, because we can do something about our posture without resorting to drugs, surgery, or other drastic measures. The way we stand, sit, and move is, to some extent, genetically laid down in terms of our skeleton's structure and the flexibility of our joints. Factors which affect our posture from birth onward include illnesses and injuries, fitness, nutrition, physical activities, and our personality and outlook on life.

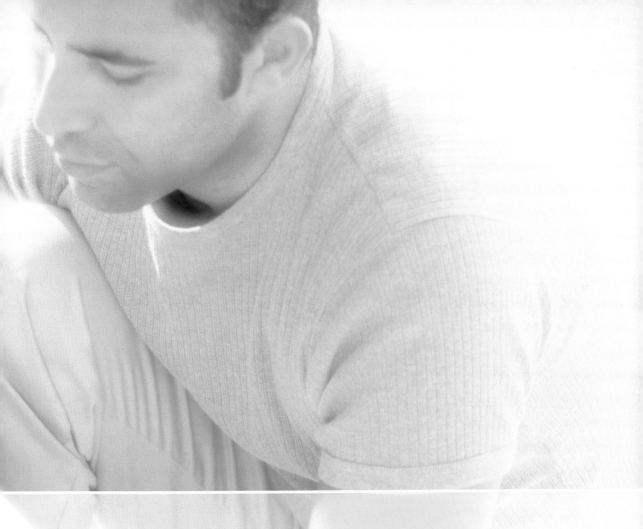

Posture that has developed over many years tends to remain fixed, but with perseverance you can alter the muscular patterns, which will bring mental as well as physical rewards. You need to think about the various muscles you use to support your spine, and the different ways in which they are brought into play.

This chapter gives detailed advice on how to improve your posture and how to make changes to your home and everyday life in order to protect your spine and prevent or improve back problems.

Standing posture

In a good standing posture, your muscles will be relaxed without being slack, and the spine itself is gently S-shaped. However, there is no single ideal posture, since people come in all shapes and sizes. The ideal posture for you is one in which your back is under the least strain, and in which the spine is curved naturally and gracefully.

The essence of good posture is fitness – if you can keep your muscles well toned and supple, you stand a good chance of achieving the correct posture for you. This is especially true if you can reinforce the posture with a relaxed mental and emotional state.

How to avoid bad posture

In the context of back pain, bad posture is one that puts your spine under unnecessary strain. Although by "poor posture" we generally mean slack posture, an excessively rigid posture can be equally bad for the back (*see below*). This results in tense muscles and may even restrict your breathing. It is not surprising that soldiers faint sometimes when they stand at attention for any length of time.

If you suffer from aching shoulders and neck, try to relax these muscles, and do not adopt a rigid stance. If you are carrying a lot of weight in front, the stress on your spine is increased, not only because your pelvis is tilted forward unnaturally

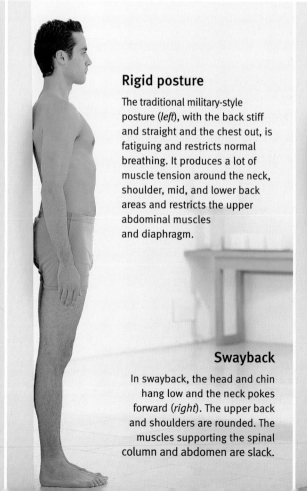

Recognizing poor posture

In one type of poor posture, the muscles are very rigid and the spine is held too stiff and straight (*near right*). In swayback posture, the muscles are too slack and the spine has exaggerated curves (*far right*). If the rigid posture looks uptight and aggressive, the swayback posture looks hangdog and submissive. Swayback is common among overweight people.

Rigid posture

The traditional military-style posture (*left*), with the back stiff and straight and the chest out, is fatiguing and restricts normal breathing. It produces a lot of muscle tension around the neck, shoulder, mid, and lower back areas and restricts the upper abdominal muscles and diaphragm.

Swayback

In swayback, the head and chin hang low and the neck pokes forward (*right*). The upper back and shoulders are rounded. The muscles supporting the spinal column and abdomen are slack.

but also because your center of gravity is moved further forward. As a consequence, the back muscles have to work harder, which increases the compression in the lower back.

It is important to strengthen your abdominal muscles and, if possible, to lose weight. If you are overweight and cannot easily go on a diet, try to increase the amount of exercise you get, perhaps by walking or cycling to work instead of driving, or climbing stairs instead of taking the elevator. Do not be tempted to use a corset – it is no substitute for getting exercise.

If you are pregnant, try to hold yourself as well as possible and make sure the surfaces where you work are adjusted to the right height (*see p. 150*), so that you do not have to stoop. Avoid wearing high heels, which can lead to a hollow back even when you are not pregnant.

Standing correctly

A major feature of the overweight or slack (sway-back) posture is that the pelvis is tilted forward, which produces a hollow back (*see left*). Try to tuck in your pelvis at every opportunity (*see right*). This movement involves consciously setting your pelvis at the correct angle so your lower back has a normal, slight curve, rather than an unnatural, hollowed-out appearance which puts the lower back under stress.

When you are busy or distracted it is easy to forget to tuck in your pelvis all the time. When you are standing, try to rest one of your feet on a low stool or foot-rail about 4 to 6in (10 to 15cm) above the floor. This relaxes the psoas muscle (*see p. 18*), which stretches from the lower back over the pelvis to the thigh, thus altering the angle between the lower back and the pelvis. You can easily use this simple technique at work and in the home and you will find that it relieves stress with no undue muscular effort.

Standing pelvic tilt

If your bad postural habits are deeply ingrained, you may find this exercise hard to begin with, but persevere. You could try it lying down at first (*see page 117*). Regularly practice the movement below and concentrate on getting the correct pelvic angle. When you can do this easily, try it without the wall and with your legs straight.

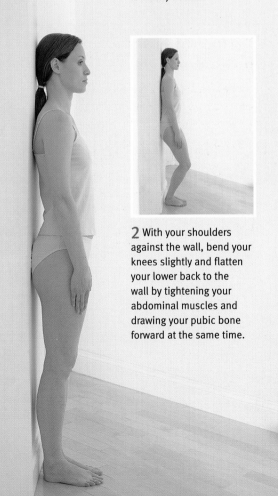

Correct pelvic angle

1 Stand with your back to a wall, so that the hollow is clearly defined.

2 With your shoulders against the wall, bend your knees slightly and flatten your lower back to the wall by tightening your abdominal muscles and drawing your pubic bone forward at the same time.

The Alexander technique

This aims to treat and prevent a range of disorders by improving posture. The technique is based on the principle of relaxing muscles – the neck and shoulder muscles particularly – and of adopting the posture that puts the least stress on your spine.

An Australian actor, F. Matthias Alexander, developed this technique after suddenly and inexplicably losing his voice during performances. He discovered that, just before delivering a speech on stage, he pulled his head backward and downward in a manner which cut off his voice. He realized that posture exerts a constant influence on both physiology and psychology.

A qualified teacher will help you undo all the postural habits that have become second nature. All pupils are taught techniques developed specifically for their own posture, which should be practiced everyday. The course may involve just five or six lessons over a few weeks or it can last up to a year.

The Alexander technique

The Alexander teacher will help you to eliminate postural defects by studying the way you sit, stand, and move. The lesson will be tailored to your unique posture. The teacher may work with you sitting, standing, or lying, depending on what she feels is required. She may start by helping you sit and stand up. You will be encouraged to imagine that you are being pulled upward from the crown of your head.

Sitting posture

The teacher will help you to achieve good sitting posture by encouraging the right amount of curve in your lower and midback and neck.

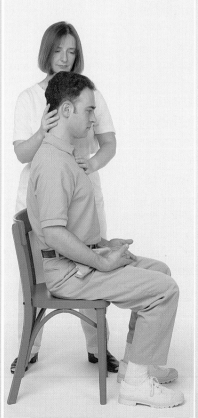

Standing up

The teacher will show you how to keep your spine straight when you stand up instead of leaning forward and pulling your head back.

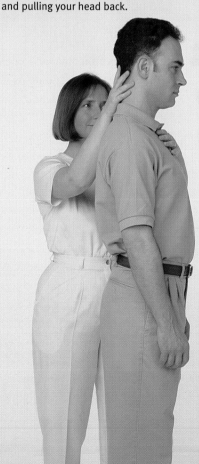

Pressure on the spine

These postures show how the pressure within the lumbar disks varies in different positions. Pressure is defined as being 100 percent when you stand up straight.

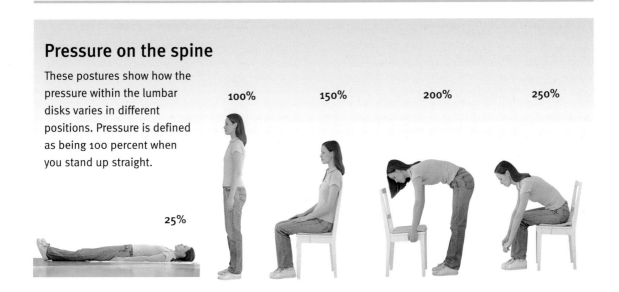

25%   100%   150%   200%   250%

A course will not cure acute problems such as a disk prolapse or stuck facet joints. However, once an acute attack is over, the technique helps to prevent a recurrence. It is especially useful for avoiding postural pain, and in elderly people it may prevent acute episodes of back pain by teaching them to use their backs properly.

Sitting posture

You increase the stress on your back if you spend long hours sitting every day. The figures above (from a chart by Alf Nachemson, an eminent researcher on back pain) tell the story.

Sitting imposes more strain on the spine than standing or walking. As soon as you lean forward more than a few degrees the pressure increases dramatically. If you must sit down for a long time, use a comfortable, well-designed chair to reduce the risk of developing either back or neck pain and a headache (*see p. 145*).

Some people find leaning forward is most comfortable for their back, providing they lean on their hands, as if riding a motorcycle. Others prefer to lean on their elbows, as when sitting on a Balans chair (*see p. 144*).

Sitting at a desk

If you work at a computer keyboard, keep your seat horizontal and support your lower back. To avoid stress in your shoulders and neck, the height of the desk or table should allow your fingers to touch the keys with your arms bent just slightly below the horizontal. Alternatively, adjust your chair to that height. For those prone to pain in the lower back, keep your chair at the correct height for the length of your legs. Sit close enough to the keyboard to work without having to stretch your arms forward from the shoulders. Finally, change position regularly and take breaks.

An ergonomically designed chair should be adjustable in height and able to tilt downward to let you lean forward and to tilt backward so you can relax. The backrest should be adjustable – the best ones tilt forward or backward according to the angle of the seat.

Head and neck alignment

If your back is rounded or you work leaning over a work surface with your head bent forward, the muscles in your upper back, shoulders, and neck can easily become fatigued. The result can be a painful neck or headaches – migraines can be induced by chronic neck tension. Whenever your neck feels tense or you hold your head forward with your chin out, reduce the curve in your neck by pulling your chin back and making the crown of your head the highest point.

The neck retraction exercise (*see p. 135*) reduces tension by bringing the weight of your head more directly over your spine, so that your neck muscles have less work to do.

Relaxing in a chair

Good sitting posture does not mean sitting up straight for long periods. You must relax in order to avoid straining muscles. Anyone attempting to sit bolt upright will, after about ten minutes, slip into a relaxed, slouched position.

The Balans chair

Originally designed in Denmark, the Balans chair (*right*) helps make you aware of your spine's position from moment to moment. Although it is almost as easy to slouch and round your lower back in this chair, you will probably be more aware that you are doing it. Obviously, this type of chair is not comfortable for people with knee problems. Even if your knees are healthy this chair takes some getting used to.

Transferring body weight

The spine should be held erect with the right amount of curve. Body weight is transferred from the pelvic bones, down the thighs and onto the knees. Ideally, the screen here should be raised to prevent neck flexion.

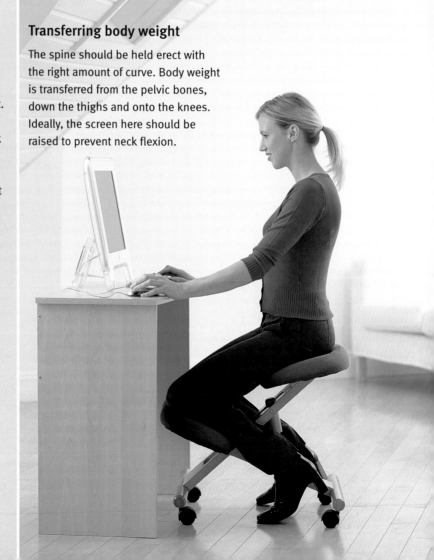

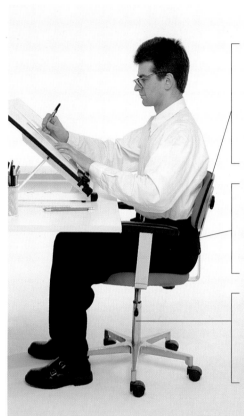

Chair back

The slight mold of the upright supports the natural arch of the lower back. Ideally, it should be high enough and broad enough to support the full width of the shoulders.

Seat depth

The seat is deep enough to support the full length to the thighs – if it were any deeper the back would be left unsupported.

Chair height

The seat is at a height that allows the feet to be firmly placed on the floor with the thighs horizontal and the lower legs perpendicular.

Choosing an appropriate chair

Anyone who spends time sitting down needs a well-designed chair which can be altered to suit their measurements. If your chair does not correspond to the ideal dimensions (*left*), either adjust it or use cushions to bring it up to the correct height or to support your back. The picture also shows the advantage of a desktop that can tilt toward you.

When you relax at home, choose a comfortable chair with enough space to let you change posture: to avoid strained, tense muscles you must be able to move around while watching television or reading. Cushions placed behind your lower back help to support your spine. Rocking chairs prevent you from sitting still for too long. The gentle motion involved is soothing and helps to relieve backache, particularly in pregnancy.

Driving

If you suffer from a bad back or from neck problems, driving a car can be an agonizing experience, unless your car is equipped with a good car seat and well-placed controls. Important factors for you to consider include: clear vision (obviously, safety has to come first); controls that are within easy reach; your arms and legs are relaxed; and your body is properly supported, especially your back.

When driving, get into the habit of relaxing your neck and shoulder muscles. Try to become aware of times when you grip the wheel too tightly or hold it too high up and with your arms outstretched. If your shoulders are hunching up toward your ears, develop a relaxed and steady breathing rhythm, and with each breath let go of the tightness in your muscles, slowly dropping your shoulders. Gently work your head and neck back into a more relaxed position against your headrest (*see p. 146*).

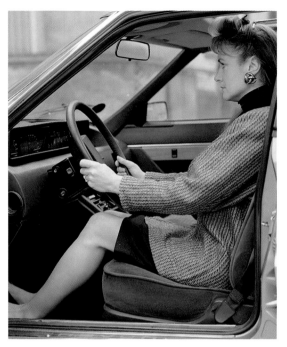

Back and head support
When driving, it is important that your back and head are adequately supported.

The car seat

The cushioning of a car seat must not slope toward the middle or too much weight will be borne by the pelvic bones instead of the thighs. The seat must be firm enough to resist the indirect forces you experience when using the pedals. If the seat is too hard, engine vibration is transmitted up to the spine, which can cause back problems.

The pedals

The pedals should not be too stiff (especially the clutch), too high off the floor, or set to one side of the driver. If you are a woman of small or average height, the foot controls may be too far apart or incorrectly angled for your feet; the strain of operating them, particularly in heavy city traffic, can lead to back pain.

The backrest

The backrest of a driver's seat should give good support to the lower back, both lengthwise and sideways. Most car seats now have an adjustable lumbar bar which you can position to suit your back. Alternatively, buy cushions for the lower back which can be attached to the backrest by a strap. If you can, alter the angle of the backrest to an optimum of between five and ten degrees behind vertical. For people, such as airline pilots, who sit in a seat for long periods, specially molded backrests can prevent back pain.

The headrest

You should be able to rest your head comfortably on the headrest, relaxing your neck and shoulder muscles, while still looking straight ahead. The headrest should be slightly padded, and adjustable both up and down, and forward and backward. The top of the headrest should be at least level with your brow at all times to effectively reduce whiplash strain (*see p. 46*).

Lying down

Many back sufferers find they are most comfortable lying down. When you lie down, you relieve your spine of much of your body's weight; this reduces the compression on a protruding disk, for example. But you don't have to lie flat: try the positions on pages 66–67 until you find the most restful one.

Your bed

If your back pain is worst in the morning, you may need to change your bed, especially if this is the only time your back aches or if this waking pain has developed only since you bought a new bed. But often aching and stiffness results from inactivity, and it may not matter which surface you lie on.

Any finely sprung mattress which supports you will do – make sure it is at least 6in (15cm) longer than you, to allow freedom of movement. Stick to what is most comfortable for you – you know best of all whether your bed is harming your back. A good mattress should be firm and provide contours for your body.

A bed base that sags or has lost its spring can harm your back. Adjustable beds are increasingly available and affordable. They can raise the legs or the head to any angle. You can also set it for the Fowler position (*see p. 66*).

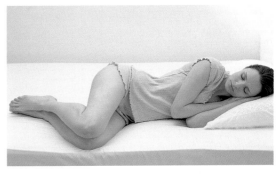

Fetal position
Some people find that lying in the fetal position brings them the most comfort and welcome relief from the pain in their back. A pillow between the knees can also be helpful.

POSITIONS TO LIE IN

Lying on your front increases the curve in the lower back and this will aggravate a backache that is caused by facet joint problems. However, this position will probably not hurt your back if your pain is caused by a prolapsed disk. See also Resting your Spine, pages 66–67.

For most people, lying flat on their backs with their legs straight out also tends to increase the curve in the lower back and cause backaches. The Fowler position, with your legs supported so that your knees are bent, helps to flatten out the excessive curve and also relaxes the psoas muscles,

Pillows

To test how good your pillow is, lift it horizontally, with the edge of your hand running across the center. If the pillow stays more or less level, all is well. If it sags, buy a new one.

If you often wake up with a stiff neck, try a pillow twisted into a butterfly shape or use a rolled and twisted towel to act as a soft collar. Or try a specially designed neck support pillow (*right*). These support your neck and prevent your head from lolling from side to side.

Neck support pillow

This pillow is ridged at the front to hold the neck and head firmly and put a very mild traction on the neck. It is divided into three sections, the two sides are slightly higher to support your head properly when you are lying on your side.

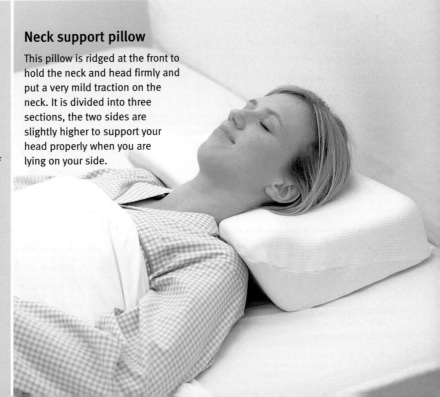

which run from the lower back to the thighs. If you have acute back pain, you may need several pillows under your knees (*see p. 66*) but otherwise a rolled-up towel may be enough.

With an adjustable bed you can raise or lower the head or the foot, relieve aching limbs and lie in a semirecumbent position if you have breathing or cardiac problems. The bed may have a vibration mode to micro-massage aching joints.

To avoid neck pain, make sure your head rests fairly square on your shoulders so the strain will be minimized. You may need one pillow if you lie on your back. If you sleep on your side, the width of your shoulders will determine whether you require one or two pillows to support your head.

Taking on jobs at work or at home

If you suffer from backache, analyze your activities at work and at home and adapt your environment accordingly. When considering your job or a task to be done at home, ask yourself the following:
- Can the effort be minimized – for example, by asking for help?
- Will you be standing awkwardly for a while?
- Does the task entail repetitive movements such as bending and twisting? If so, work only for short periods at a time, with intervals of rest in between.
- Is the task too strenuous for you?
- Can you lift and carry things properly?

Lifting techniques

When you lift anything, avoid bending your back. Always take the weight on your leg muscles. When putting the object down, reverse this sequence.

Lifting a box

1 Squat down on your haunches with one foot slightly in front of the other and the object between your knees. Grasp the object firmly with your hands – place one hand under it with that arm straight, and steady it with the other arm.

2 Keep your back straight and lean forward slightly. Stand up in one smooth motion, keeping the object close to you and taking the weight on your legs. Do not bend your back as you stand up.

3 When you carry an object, always keep its weight close to your body.

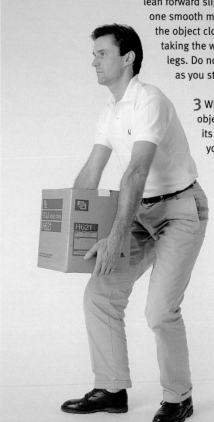

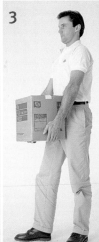

3

- Does the task involve constant postural stress – for example, as in painting a ceiling?
- Is there repetitive stress involved – for example, driving heavy vehicles over rough, bumpy road?

If you decide the job is feasible, plan it out with the following guidelines:

- Above all, concentrate on the job. If your mind is distracted, or you are under pressure, the risk of back injury increases.
- Try to anticipate pitfalls before starting the job.
- Wear appropriate clothing: nice clothes may make you hold objects away from your body, putting extra stress on your back.
- Make sure you can stand properly with adequate space around you and without stooping.

- Lift and handle objects carefully (*see below*).
- Lean with your back against heavy objects to move them, instead of pushing with your arms.
- Buy any tools needed to make the task easier.
- Avoid unnecessary effort: put objects on a suitable work surface to avoid stooping; use a cart or other device to save effort. If you can lift the object easily with one hand, use the other to provide support and stability.
- Divide a big load into smaller loads. If you can't, leave it. When traveling or shopping, divide your suitcases or purchases evenly into two loads.
- Let other parts of the body, such as shoulders, pelvis, or thighs, take the weight.
- Drop objects that are not fragile.

Lifting a long load

1 Squat down with one leg in front of the other and one end of the load between your feet. Put both hands under the end nearest to you.

2 Lift one end of the load until it is vertical, and rest it against your shoulder. Shift one hand if necessary to prevent the load toppling over.

3 Grip the load firmly underneath with your other hand. Stand up, keeping your back straight, and taking the weight with your legs.

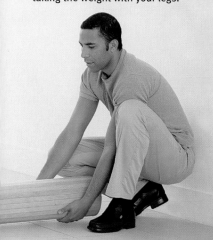

2

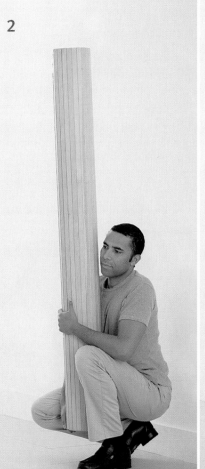

3

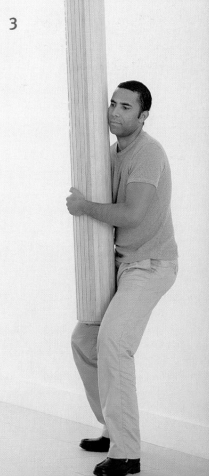

House and garden work

Much of the work involved in running a house is stressful for back sufferers, but you can reduce the stresses and strains with the following adaptations to your home and careful planning of tasks.

• **Kitchen** An ergonomically designed kitchen will pay dividends. For most jobs, a countertop should be slightly lower than your elbow (*see below*). The sink needs to be at elbow height to avoid stooping when washing dishes. When standing at a sink or countertop, rest one foot on a low stool or foot rail.

• **Bathroom** To shave, use a mirror at one side of the sink or an extendable mirror. When washing your hair, kneel down by the bath and use a shower hose. When bathing, avoid lying with your back in a rounded position for too long – getting out may be hard. Attach a handrail to the bath if you have chronic back trouble, or use the shower.

• **Washing clothes** Put the basket on a low chair before emptying the washing machine. Keep the clothes line at a sensible height to avoid straining.

• **Ironing** Make sure the ironing board is at the right height (*see below*) to avoid stooping.

• **Bed making** Buy fitted sheets and comforters. Squat down or kneel by the bed when you tuck in the sheets. Install smooth-running casters.

• **Cleaning** Use long-handled implements and, where possible, kneel down to clean. Keep your spine straight instead of bending from the waist.

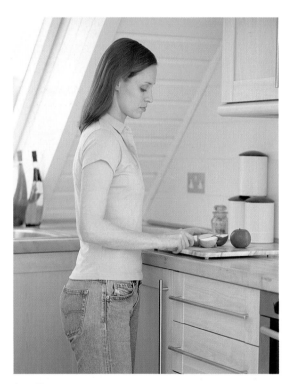

Standing at a countertop
The countertop should be 2 to 3in (5 to 7cm) lower than your elbow, so that you do not stoop over it. Stand as close as possible to it, and rest your hips against it.

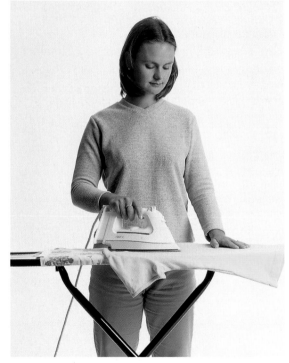

Ironing clothes
The ironing board should be low enough so that you do not have to bend your elbow at an angle of less than 90 degrees but high enough that you do not have to stoop.

Working in the garden

Many garden tasks involve crouching, bending, or lifting. Try to work in an upright position, follow the lifting rules (*see pp. 148–49*) and change tasks often.

Work with good tools. If you can, use long-handled tools and kneel down to work. You could convert your garden to raised beds or grow plants in a greenhouse.

Shoveling earth

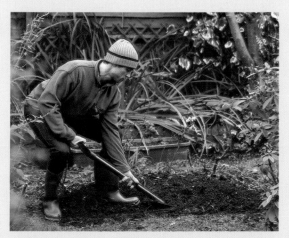

1 Keep your back as straight as possible and your knees bent. Slide the shovel along the ground, resting the back of your top hand against the inside of your knee or thigh.

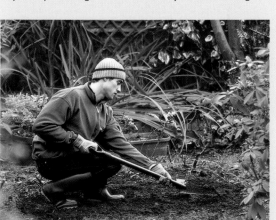

2 When you have a spadeful, throw the soil to one side using a sideways movement, instead of lifting it first. Avoid using wheelbarrows because they are usually badly designed for backs and don't dig when the soil is wet and heavy or hard, dry, and compacted.

Digging in the garden

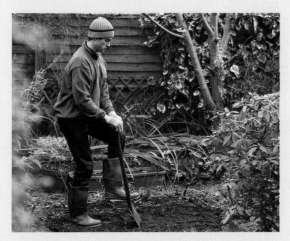

1 Don't grip the spade too tightly and work at a steady pace. Push the spade into the ground using your body weight, not your muscle power.

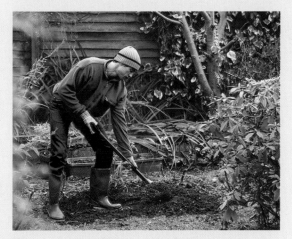

2 Cut around the sides of each spadeful before you start to lift the soil. Hold the handle at the end and use the spade as a lever to ease out the soil. Lift the soil by holding the shaft of the spade near its base. Do not lift too much at one time, and turn it over as soon as you can.

Caring for children

Taking care of young children involves lifting, carrying, and stooping over beds. Pay special attention to the way you lift and watch for unexpected problems such as children who struggle when being picked up.

Children are not the sole cause of back trouble, but they certainly constitute a risk, especially for women – it takes up to five months for the ligaments of the spine and pelvis to tighten up again after the birth. So if you are a new mother, you will be particularly vulnerable to developing back strain from weak and overstretched stomach muscles, poor posture, or faulty lifting.

Choose a crib with a side that can be lowered right down since this saves you from bending over in an awkward position to pick up your baby.

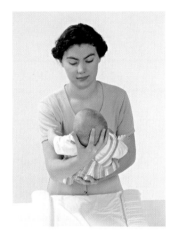

Washing and changing a baby
You can do these jobs on a work surface a little below elbow level, such as a chest of drawers. Or you can kneel on the floor and change your baby on a low bed or sofa.

Whenever you can, carry your baby in a special baby carrier on your back to distribute his weight close to your center of gravity. Slings worn at the front tend to slacken and impose a strain similar to that of pregnancy, except the baby is heavier now.

Lifting a child

When you lift a child, follow the basic rules of lifting: squat down by the child and use your leg muscles to rise up again, keeping your back straight as you stand up.

Squatting down

Before you pick up your child, squat down with one foot firmly on the floor. Keeping your back straight, lift your child with both hands under her shoulders.

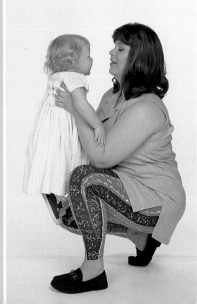

Standing up

As you stand up, let your strong leg muscles bear the load.

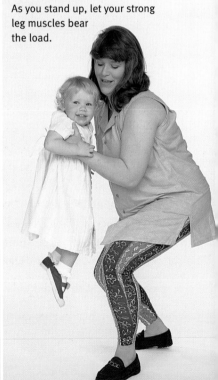

Sports

It is difficult to identify which sports are more likely to expose you to the risk of back problems. However, certain movements or activities may aggravate existing problems. If you are prone to recurrent backaches, be alert for sharp twinges or an intermittent ache. When you notice them, avoid sports such as golf or soccer, which involve vigorous twisting, turning, or bending, and redouble your preventative exercises.

Warming up and cooling down

You must always warm up before any sport: cycle for five to ten minutes on an exercise machine, jog on the spot for a similar period or follow the "patter" routine – keep your toes on the ground and lift the heels alternately as rapidly as possible, raising your knees a little each time. Once your pulse rate increases a little, perform muscle-stretching exercises appropriate to your sport for another five or ten minutes. After vigorous exercise you should cool down, repeating the stretches you did at the start.

High risk sports

You can reduce the risk of injuring your spine in certain sports if you keep particular muscle groups in good shape. Golfers need good muscular support, particularly from the muscles which run down and across the abdomen. Serving in tennis or badminton and bowling can stress the facet joints in the lower spine. To avoid problems, try muscle-strengthening exercises (*see p. 124*).

Long-distance running stresses the lower body's joints. Regular stretching of hamstrings and lower back muscles helps avoid problems. Check, too, on the angle of your pelvic tilt (*see p. 141*), wear well-cushioned running shoes and, as you run, avoid swinging your arms across your front too much.

General fitness

Fitness is important for everyone, not only for people who play sports. If you are fit, then a good, relaxed posture probably comes naturally. If you have recurring back pain caused by poor posture, take up exercises to make you fit, once an episode of acute pain has died down. You will then be less likely to injure yourself; and if you do, the damage will probably be less severe, and your general fitness will help you recover more quickly.

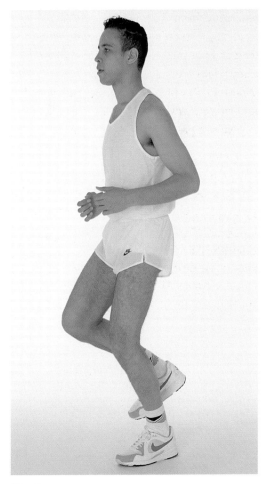

Warming up
Before doing any sports it is essential that you spend time exercising to warm yourself up.

Coping
with Chronic Pain

Severe or prolonged pain can result in dramatic changes of behavior and mood which, in turn, can affect the intensity of the pain and the sufferer's ability to tolerate it. Recently, we have begun to understand the neurophysiological and chemical changes that underlie these psychological effects and signal the transition from a relatively simple pain problem into "chronic pain disorder." Often, there are bizzare feelings that doctors cannot explain: abnormal burning, drawing sensations; exquisite sensitivity of the skin to gentle touch or

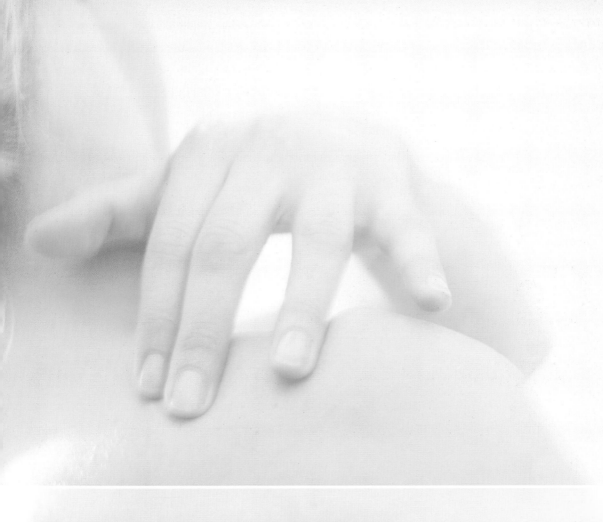

pressure; prolonged aftereffects to either movement or exercise; hot and cold sensations; and trickling or crawling sensations down the legs.

Because there is effectively no medical cure for chronic pain disorder, psychological and functional rehabilitation is extremely important. If you have been in pain for months or years, your entire nervous system and personality will be affected. You need to learn to see the whole picture of your pain disorder, so that you can minimize its effects and live as full and enjoyable a life as possible.

Pain perception

We are only just beginning to understand the psychology of pain perception. The amount of pain you feel depends not only on the physical damage, but also on your mental state. You can be unaware of some slight injury if your mind is occupied with something else. At the other extreme, there are reports of people feeling pain in an amputated limb.

GATE CONTROL THEORY

Two renowned neurologists, Ronald Melzack and Patrick Wall, developed the gate control theory of pain perception. They visualized mental and physical factors opening or closing a "gate," controlling the amount of pain that can be felt. Normally, the gate is closed and no pain is felt, but when there is an injury, various factors battle to push the gate open or to close it again. The pain's intensity depends on how wide the gate is open.

The pain gate

This diagram shows how the pain gate is opened and closed by opposing factors, and how the pain message can be blocked even after the T-cell, which starts a chain reaction, has been triggered.

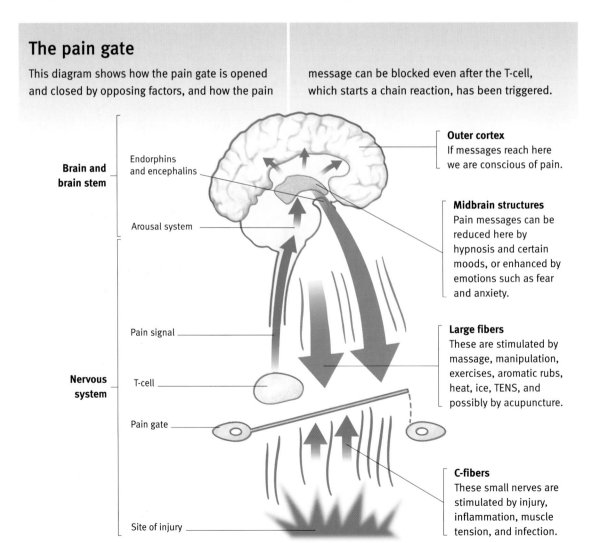

Brain and brain stem

Endorphins and encephalins

Arousal system

Outer cortex
If messages reach here we are conscious of pain.

Midbrain structures
Pain messages can be reduced here by hypnosis and certain moods, or enhanced by emotions such as fear and anxiety.

Pain signal

Nervous system

T-cell

Pain gate

Large fibers
These are stimulated by massage, manipulation, exercises, aromatic rubs, heat, ice, TENS, and possibly by acupuncture.

Site of injury

C-fibers
These small nerves are stimulated by injury, inflammation, muscle tension, and infection.

Factors affecting pain perception

Susceptibility to pain is greater when the brain is highly active or when the arousal system is inactive. Decreased brain activity and increased arousal system activity both dull the intensity of pain. The mental and physical states listed below influence the perception of pain. Some of these states decrease or dull the intensity of pain while others exaggerate or increase it.

Decrease pain

- Emotional tranquillity
- Sleep
- Hypnosis
- Hyperventilation (which causes reduced carbon dioxide)
- Excess alcohol
- Focusing on activities to distract the mind
- Increase in adrenalin
- Drugs such as valium and morphine

Increase pain

- Anxiety and uncertainty
- Fear
- Depression
- Concentrating attention on pain
- Drinking small amounts of tea, coffee, and alcohol
- Drugs such as amphetamines and barbiturates

Neural impulses

The pain gate is pushed open by small C-fiber nerves which relay pain messages from the site of the injury or inflammation. Massage, rubs, and other therapies stimulate larger fibers and help to close the gate again, reducing the intensity of the pain. If small-fiber messages swamp those from large fibers, the gate opens and a cell known as a T-cell is triggered, which starts a chain reaction through the nervous system, the brain stem, and the center of the brain to the outer cortex, where it is registered as a conscious perception of pain. At any stage, the pain messages can be blocked.

Arousal system activity

The brain stem controls nervous functions known collectively as the arousal system. When your mind is calm or sedated by drugs such as valium, this system is active and pain messages are muted before they reach the brain. The system is less active when the brain is highly active – with worry or fear, for example – and when you take drugs such as barbiturates. In these states, the pain is more intense.

Pain-reducing hormones

The brain itself can also close the pain gate. Before you consciously feel any pain, the brain stimulates the production of encephalins and endorphins which help to reduce your perception of pain. Drugs such as morphine and valium supplement the endorphins. Acupuncture may also control pain by encouraging the production of endorphins and by stimulating the large fibers.

MENTAL ATTITUDES

Pain messages can be blocked or reduced between the center of the brain and the outer cortex. Your general state of mind, including your expectations, anxieties, mood, will to recover, and ability to concentrate on something else, is the decisive factor. Pain control therapies such as hypnosis and the placebo effect probably block messages at this stage. The mind, in effect, has an arsenal of weapons, conscious and subconscious, which can work to subdue or increase the level of pain.

Motivation

Inevitably, not everyone is equally motivated to recover quickly from a back problem. People with an enjoyable social life or a rewarding job will be eager to return to normal, and this will speed up their recovery.

Others may welcome the extra attention and sympathy they get from being ill. There may be rewards, such as a sick pay worker's compensation or litigation. These people may take longer to recover. Measures apparently unrelated to their back condition, such as changing jobs or taking on different duties at work, may hasten their recovery.

The effect on others

Your pain may affect the mood and behavior of people around you, in much the same way as it affects you. People caring for you can be just as worried and depressed by your pain as you are. The best way of caring for someone suffering from chronic pain is to encourage as much normal activity and independence as possible, while remaining sympathetic and making allowances for the person's pain and disability.

Your disability may have a serious effect on your partner, particularly if he or she is carrying you or helping you with basics such as feeding, washing, or dressing. It is worthwhile to explore your reactions to the new situation together. The extra work thrown on to your partner by your disability may make you feel guilty and, at the same time, make your partner feel resentful.

Coping with pain

Most people with long-term back pain experience emotional and psychological problems they have not previously encountered and are not trained to handle. If your condition is unlikely to improve with further treatment, you should seek help for coping with long-term pain. But be realistic and avoid disappointment or a sense of failure.

If your pain does not disappear, try to diminish its impact on your life and find ways of decreasing the pain itself. Therapies to help you cope with pain can succeed only if you participate actively. Techniques such as meditation and relaxation can teach you ways of helping yourself to change self-defeating patterns of thought and behavior, and to adapt to a new lifestyle.

Acupuncture

The goal of the ancient Chinese art of acupuncture is twofold: first, to identify the imbalance of energy which is causing a disease; and second, to alter the energy flow until a harmonious balance is restored. In general, acupuncture helps most back problems by reducing muscle tension and thereby relieving pain and improving mobility.

You are not guaranteed relief even if you have a condition of the spine that is potentially amenable to acupuncture (*see right*). It depends on how you respond. Good responders do not have to believe in the treatment – they are decisive, impulsive, artistically or creatively inclined, and ready to take risks. Poor responders are the opposite.

Trigger point needling

One exciting discovery in acupuncture is trigger point needling, or intramuscular stimulation. Acupuncture needles are inserted into trigger

Which conditions respond best to acupuncture?

We are beginning to understand more about how best to use acupuncture and what kind of back pain it helps most. In the meantime, if you have any of the problems listed here, and if other treatments have not stopped your pain, acupuncture is well worth trying. As long as the treatment is given by a well-qualified practitioner, acupuncture will certainly not be harmful. In so far as it is possible, I will attempt to list the conditions that may benefit from acupuncture.

Most likely to respond

- Acute low back pain and acute torticollis – whether caused by a disk protrusion or facet joint problem
- Wear and tear (osteoarthritis) of the facet joints
- Episodes of acute pain due to instability in the lower back
- Trigger point pain

Reasonably likely

- Mild sciatica without signs of damage to the nerve root such as weakness or numbness
- Sacroiliac strain

Somewhat less likely

- Agonizing sciatica with definite signs of nerve root damage
- Severe cervical radiculopathy

Not to be considered

- Central disk prolapse with sciatica in both legs, or bladder or bowel disturbance

The meridians

To an acupuncturist energy flows through the body along a network of channels called meridians. Each meridian relates to a major organ and its functions. Meridians are of different lengths and each has a number of influential points along it. For example, the heart meridian runs from the armpit to the fingertip and has nine acupuncture points. The bladder meridian runs from the forehead, around the back of the skull, down the back, and along the leg to the foot. It has 67 acupuncture points.

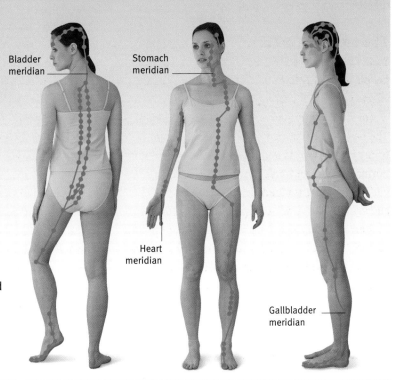

Bladder meridian

Stomach meridian

Heart meridian

Gallbladder meridian

points (*see p. 48*) – hypersensitive areas usually found within taut bands of muscle that lie along the spine – bringing relief from long-standing pain and improvements in mobility.

CONSULTING AN ACUPUNCTURIST

An acupuncturist may help at any stage in your back condition, although it is always wise to have a medical diagnosis first. Most people will have tried, or will have been offered, the more conventional therapies and may consider an acupuncturist:

- When rest, physical therapy, manipulation, or analgesics are not helping to resolve an acute episode of pain.
- To reduce pain and inflammation arising from

osteoarthritis in the facet joints which do not respond to improved posture, exercises, or traction; or as an alternative to local injections to the joints or prolotherapy (*see p. 101*).

- When chronic back pain or sciatica is not amenable to surgery, has failed to be relieved by surgery, or for which the patient has declined surgery. Acupuncture may help in certain conditions such as trigger points (*see p. 48*).
- When chronic "pain patterns" have set in. Acupuncture may help to break the vicious cycle, perhaps by helping to close the pain gate.

My advice is to choose an acupuncturist who has a thorough background, training and experience, but who is also medically qualified.

Consulting an acupuncturist

On your first visit, an acupuncturist will take a detailed case history of your symptoms and ask you about such things as your reaction to changes in the weather, and your food and drink preferences. The acupuncturist will take your pulse and look at your tongue and complexion before deciding on a treatment. She may occasionally use smoldering moxa to clear blocked channels and reestablish the flow of energy.

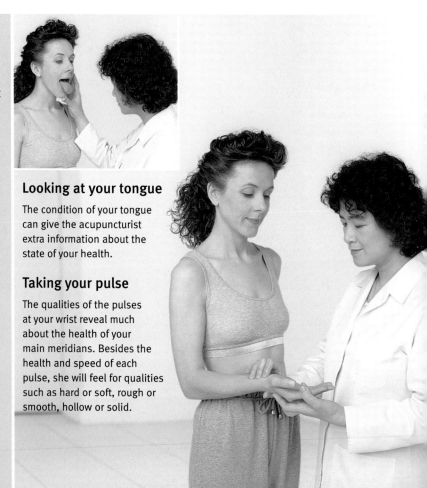

Looking at your tongue

The condition of your tongue can give the acupuncturist extra information about the state of your health.

Taking your pulse

The qualities of the pulses at your wrist reveal much about the health of your main meridians. Besides the health and speed of each pulse, she will feel for qualities such as hard or soft, rough or smooth, hollow or solid.

Meditation

Regular meditation can help you recognize and reduce stress in your body, and to overcome the anxieties and fears that cause it. People in chronic pain and back sufferers whose muscles are chronically tense and who are very anxious are particular beneficiaries.

Meditation aims to bring the mind under control and focus it in such a way that you are freed from stressful fears and emotions. It can also lower the heart beat and respiration rate. By synchronizing and harmonizing the electrical patterns from the brain, it can induce alpha brainwaves, which generally indicate calmness.

Types of meditation

Initially, it is easier to learn meditation from a teacher. Look for a local center or group who will teach you the basic techniques; some family physicians run meditation groups in their practices and centers. If no teacher is accessible, try the meditation on pages 162–163.

The type of meditation most appropriate for you depends partly on your personality and the state of your back, and partly on personal choice. The active forms of meditation, of which Rajneesh is the best known, involve spontaneous movement, adopting various postures, deep breathing, and facial contortions. If you have recurrent back pain that is partly the result of postural tension, this

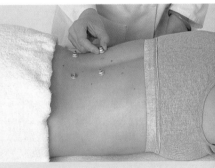

Receiving treatment

As you lie on a couch the acupuncturist inserts sterilized acupuncture needles into particular points on your body. This may be painless or create a fine, stinging sensation that lasts for a second or two. The acupuncturist will then leave you to relax for 10 to 15 minutes.

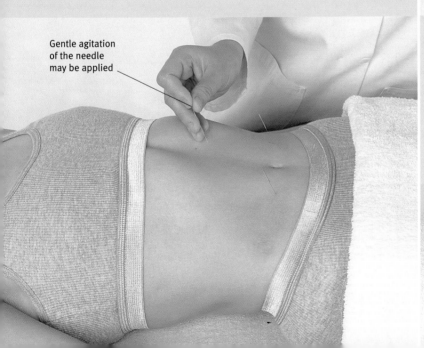

Gentle agitation of the needle may be applied

Treatment with moxibustion

The acupuncturist may insert needles into the relevant points and burn small cones of wormword over them. Card disks around the base will catch the ash (*above*). Alternatively, the acupuncturist may hold a lighted moxa roll over the acupuncture point to heat it (*below*).

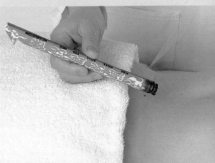

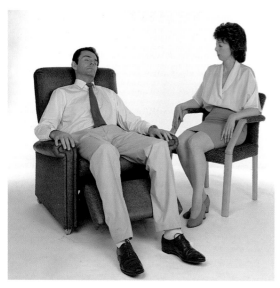

Hypnotherapy
A hypnotist can help you access the subconscious functions of your brain, giving you the power to control your perception of pain.

may help you to loosen up, emotionally and physically. But it may not be the best choice if you have an acutely painful back.

The more passive forms of meditation include transcendental, Buddhist, and yoga techniques. In the first, you raise your consciousness by silently and rhythmically repeating a word or sound. Yoga or Buddhist meditation combines breathing with concentration on a single object or thought.

Hypnotherapy

Hypnotherapy helps you influence your perception of pain. Under hypnosis, your control over your conscious mind is suspended temporarily, so that your subconscious thoughts, feelings, and memories can be reached. Even when you come out of the hypnotic trance and are fully conscious, the pain will be considerably reduced.

Not all people respond equally well. People who can let go, trust others, and relax are the best responders. You, as the patient, must be willing to accept the ideas presented by the hypnotist. If you do not respond effectively to hypnotherapy, you may still benefit from a form of self-hypnosis.

Relaxation

Learning a relaxation technique reduces your pain by giving you greater conscious control over your body. You become aware of tension and stress and can release particularly tense muscles. Relaxation also influences the arousal system (*see p. 157*), and this may underlie the feeling of improvement.

Simple meditation method

Choose a quiet room without distracting noises such as television, radio, or music. Sit or lie down in whichever position you find the most effortless and comfortable. Put a folded towel under your knees and a pillow under your head. Start by closing your eyes and relaxing all your muscles. Don't worry about how deeply you relax; this will come with time and practice. Worrying about it will probably tense you up anyway.

EMG (electromyographic) feedback

One relaxation method uses EMG feedback: sensors placed on particular groups of muscles, usually around the neck and shoulder area or on the lower back, are attached to a small machine which emits a signal – a click or a flashing light. The tenser the muscles, the faster the signal. You lie down during your first sessions with a therapist; later, you can use the machine as you sit, stand, or walk. You may be able to use the machine at home.

Other relaxation methods

Autogenic training, contract-relax, and meditation (*see p. 161*) are techniques you can learn from a trained therapist or from tape-recorded lessons.

Autogenic training is a form of autosuggestion or self-hypnosis, in which you repeat certain phrases instructing various muscle areas to relax. Regularly repeating these verbal cues can enable you to relax quickly and at will.

Contract-relax encourages you to recognize the difference between tensing your muscles briefly but strongly, and then relaxing them completely. The sudden change from one to the other enhances awareness of how much tension is in your muscles.

In some respects the EMG machine provides a shortcut to the more traditional methods by providing you automatically with information about the tension in your body. If you have been in chronic pain for several months, you may not be

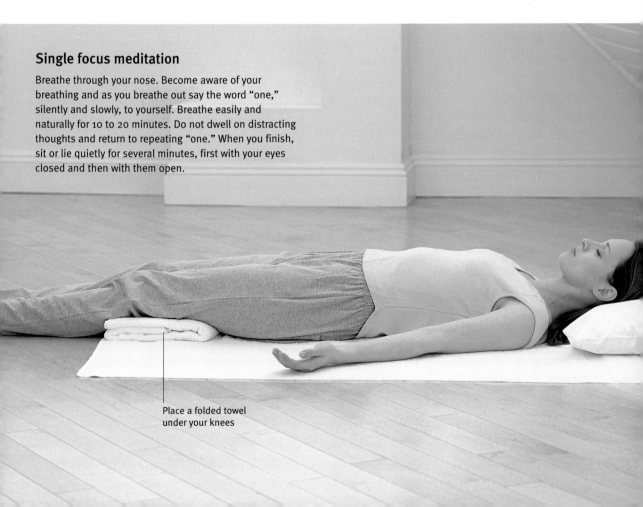

Single focus meditation

Breathe through your nose. Become aware of your breathing and as you breathe out say the word "one," silently and slowly, to yourself. Breathe easily and naturally for 10 to 20 minutes. Do not dwell on distracting thoughts and return to repeating "one." When you finish, sit or lie quietly for several minutes, first with your eyes closed and then with them open.

Place a folded towel under your knees

aware of how tense your muscles have become, so the direct feedback from an EMG machine could be useful before you practice any of the other methods given here.

The success of these methods is influenced greatly by the result of the initial session. For example, if pain has disturbed your sleep for several days and you sleep soundly after the first relaxation session, subsequent sessions are likely to be successful, too. In addition, you can keep a record of the level of pain you experience before and after relaxation sessions: any improvement will encourage you to continue.

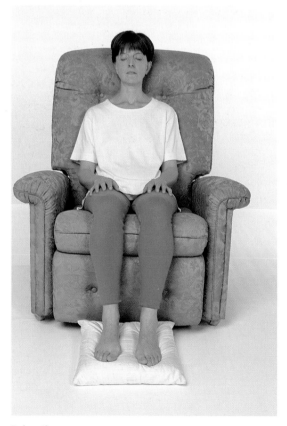

Relaxation
Relax in a comfortable chair with your back straight and your feet on a soft pillow so your thighs are horizontal.

Tackling your mood

Certain moods, such as depression and anxiety, can heighten your sensitivity to pain and delay recovery. Both can be caused by chronic pain in the first place, so a vicious circle easily develops. It is therefore extremely important to recognize these moods in yourself and try to overcome them.

Depression

As a medical term, depression means more than simple unhappiness because it includes physical changes as well. If you have most or all of the following symptoms, you should seek professional help for depression:

- Reduced or greatly increased appetite and weight
- Marked changes of mood
- Lethargy and listlessness
- Inability to enjoy any pastime
- Disturbed sleep.

One way to minimize or prevent depression is to focus on the clear physical source of your pain, but doctors and other practitioners often prescribe drugs to treat depression. The drugs traditionally used are called "tricyclics." It may be two or three weeks before you notice any effect. Try to follow your doctor's instructions precisely and take the full course. Tricyclics are not addictive but they may make you feel drowsy. Rarely, they make your heart race and your mouth dry. You may also have difficulty urinating and your vision might become blurred.

Serotonin is an important brain chemical that becomes depleted during depression. The way Prozac and other modern antidepressants work is by counteracting this depletion, helping to level out mood. They also have fewer side effects.

Many patients with chronic nerve pain or muscle pain (such as fibromyalgia) are prescribed a drug called amitriptyline in a low dose of 25mg, about a sixth of the usual antidepressant dose. This is not given for depression – it is intended to directly stimulate the "descending inhibitory pathways," which are the nerves that act to block the central transmission of pain. Amitriptyline is especially useful for back pain sufferers because, if it is taken at night, it can improve your quality of sleep – another important factor in coping with chronic pain.

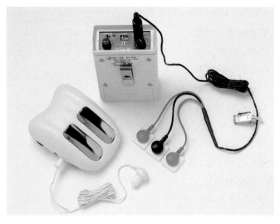

Portable sensors
The muscle biofeedback unit (*top*) and the galvanic skin response sensor (*left*) are two biofeedback devices that you can take with you wherever you go.

Anxiety

People suffering from chronic pain often become very anxious, without necessarily having a definite cause. Tranquilizers such as valium can calm you

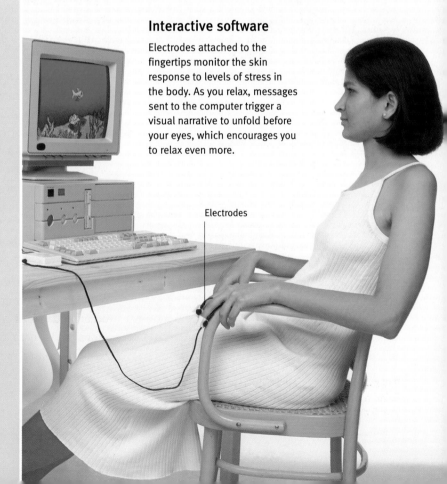

Biofeedback equipment

Several types of machine are available that can feed back information about various body functions, including brainwave patterns, electrical skin resistance, and muscle tension.

Interactive software

Electrodes attached to the fingertips monitor the skin response to levels of stress in the body. As you relax, messages sent to the computer trigger a visual narrative to unfold before your eyes, which encourages you to relax even more.

Electrodes

are severely disabling, both for the patients and for their surrounding family. Some drugs, such as imipramine (a tricyclic antidepressant), can block or prevent these panic attacks.

Reducing pain behavior

People who have failed to improve with all the tried-and-tested approaches, and are suffering chronic pain, may spiral downward in a vicious cycle of pain, despair, inactivity, and disability. A multimodal approach is necessary. Modern drugs such as carbamazepine and gabapentin, TENS (*see p. 169*), or acupuncture may be tried if they have not been used so far. Morphine-type drugs, such as tramadol, buprenorphine, and fentanyl patches, can be given to control severe pain with minimum side effects. Addiction is not an issue here.

A rehabilitation program combined with psychological help can benefit those who exhibit increased pain behavior and the resulting disability. They will be encouraged to focus on function instead of the pain, its causes, seeking a magic cure, or the secondary gain of attention and sympathy from carergivers. This is a gradual process undertaken with a group of sufferers in a caring environment with input from psychologists, pain specialists, physical therapists, and nurses. Enormous gains can be made and many patients are enabled to turn their whole life around.

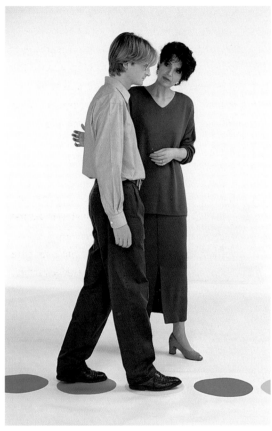

Neurolinguistic programming (NLP)
This psychotherapeutic technique can help a patient "reframe" the way they respond to their pain and set them on a new and more positive pathway.

down, especially if something specific is worrying you. However, these drugs cannot be used over a long time – they are addictive and do not help you to overcome your anxiety. Never harbor hidden fears about your illness since it only adds to your stress. Always discuss such fears with your doctor.

Some people experience severe panic attacks, isolated episodes approaching extreme terror, accompanied by a variety of physical symptoms such as palpitations, pains in the chest, shortness of breath, and panting. A few develop phobias such as agoraphobia. Naturally, these complications

Defeating insomnia

Adaptive response training can be used to help cure the insomnia which plagues many people with chronic back pain. The therapy encourages you to tackle your sleep problem head on, instead of letting your pain rule your sleeping habits. It's designed to to establish routines conducive to a normal sleep pattern. The basic instructions include:

- Only lie down to sleep when you feel sleepy.
- Do not do anything (except for sexual activity) in bed except sleep.
- If you do not fall asleep within 15 minutes of getting into bed, get up and leave the bedroom. Do not return to bed until you are sleepy.
- Set the alarm for the same time every morning. Get up regardless of how much sleep you've had.
- Avoid daytime naps.
- Avoid coffee, tea, and other stimulants.

Cognitive behavioral therapy (CBT)

CBT is a practical, humanistic therapy that focuses on the present and advises against dwelling on the past. You and your therapist will uncover and examine any negative thought patterns and irrational fears and work together to break these unhealthy patterns. The emphasis is on learning to cope, and developing strategies to help you do this – accepting your present limitations and working constructively with them. Gradually you will regain control of the pain, your body and your life.

Neurostimulation

Many pain clinics offer this technique to alleviate both acute and chronic pain. Electrical stimulation probably reduces pain, at least in part, by stimulating the large fibers that close the pain gate (*see p. 156*) and interrupt the pain messages from

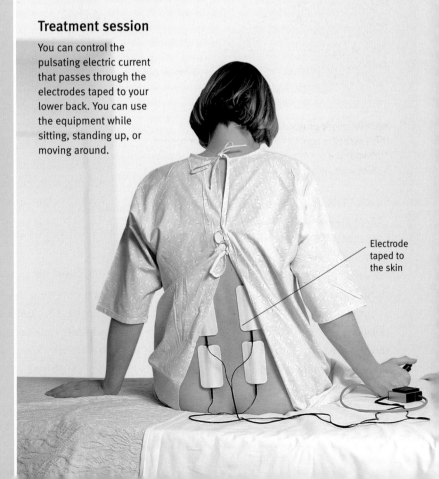

Transcutaneous nerve stimulation

A pulsating current is passed through electrodes which are placed on your skin. The rate of the pulse and the voltage can be varied according to the nature of your pain. Though this treatment is safe enough to be used at home, you should never place the electrodes anywhere near the carotid artery in your neck.

Treatment session

You can control the pulsating electric current that passes through the electrodes taped to your lower back. You can use the equipment while sitting, standing up, or moving around.

Electrode taped to the skin

Implanted stimulators

Minute electrodes are implanted in the spinal canal and connected to a tiny generator by subcutaneous wires. This picture shows where electrodes are placed for nerve damage pain in the legs or for pain associated with the sympathetic nervous system. For angina or heart pain they would be implanted higher; for arm pain they would need to be in the neck.

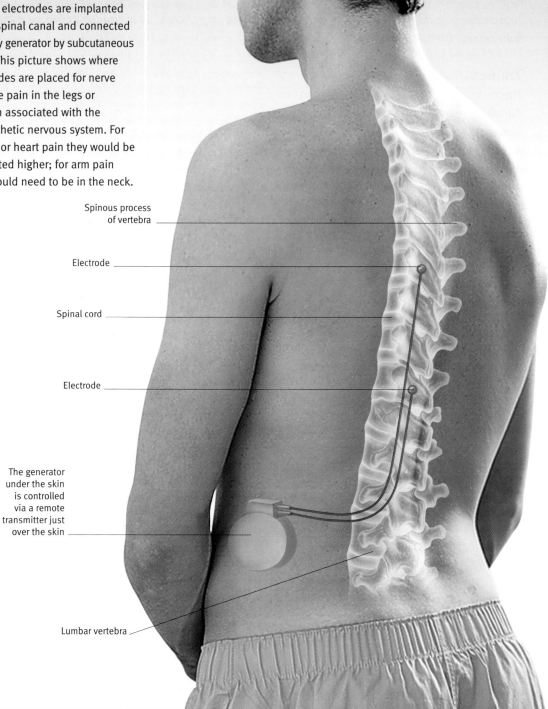

Spinous process of vertebra

Electrode

Spinal cord

Electrode

The generator under the skin is controlled via a remote transmitter just over the skin

Lumbar vertebra

C-fibers. It increases the level of the body's pain inhibiting hormones, the endorphins and encephalins, which circulate in the cerebro-spinal fluid bathing the nerves in the spinal canal.

Transcutaneous stimulation (TENS)

This treatment is the most common method of stimulating nerves electrically. The method is safe, though there are certain restrictions for people with cardiac pacemakers or who are in the first three months of pregnancy.

About 50 percent of patients find that TENS treatment reduces their pain. Some have somewhat short-lived relief, but experience continuing benefit from using the machine in the long term. One advantage of TENS is that it reduces the need for analgesics and narcotics. These drugs may be effective in dealing with acute pain, but in the long term they suppress the body's ability to produce endorphins and encephalins.

Implanted neurostimulators

If the pain is severe enough, nerves can be stimulated very effectively by a neurostimulator implanted in the spinal cord. Less common than TENS, this treatment is restricted to cases where back surgery has failed. It is particularly useful for people with irreparably damaged nerves. Between 50 and 60 percent of users benefit from an epidural nerve stimulation system. It is best used intermittently rather than continuously, because this increases the production of natural pain-reducing hormones.

This implant does not completely relieve the pain – you will still feel any sharply localized pain. The implant blocks pain by stimulating the large fibers which close the pain gate (*see p. 156*). It has the further advantage of increasing the blood flow to a formerly painful extremity by dilating the blood vessels. This is particularly helpful for the diffuse burning pain caused by damage to the sympathetic nerves. An implant can even heal ulcers caused by poor circulation.

People who remain on narcotic medicines after an implant often feel the electrical sensation of stimulation, but obtain no pain relief from it. Their pain can be reduced by taking certain nutritional supplements and antidepressant drugs, which increase production of the body's own pain-reducing hormones.

Other spinal implants

People with so-called "failed back" syndrome are now increasingly being given other forms of spinal implant. These include epidural catheters with continuous infusion of local anesthetic for up to a week to allow active rehabilitation. In some centers the catheters are implanted for 120 days and the patient controls the infusion rate at home for a "pain vacation."

Opiates can also be given via a slow-release system implanted under the skin at much lower doses than you would have to use by mouth and therefore with fewer side effects and minimal risk of addiction. These can be used in the long term for those with severe uncontrollable pain.

Deep brain stimulators

A few people with very severe and widespread pain are treated with a stimulating electrode implanted deep in the brain that appears to encourage production of endorphins and encephalins. Since there is a slight risk of brain damage, this operation is performed only in extreme cases.

Present research aims to develop devices that can switch on and off according to the levels of hormones circulating in the blood. Such devices will respond automatically to the body's needs.

Useful addresses

United States

AARP National Headquarters
601 E Street, NW A9
Washington, DC 20049
Tel: (202) 434-2560
www.aarp.org

AliMed Inc.
297 High Street
Dedham, MA 02026
Tel: (800) 225-2610
Tel: (781) 329-2900
info@alimed.com

American Academy of Medical Acupuncture
4929 Wilshire Blvd., Suite 428
Los Angeles, CA 90010
Tel: (323) 937-5514
JDOWDEN@prodigy.net

American Back Society
St. Joseph's Professional Center
2647 International Blvd.,
Suite 401
Oakland, CA 94601
Tel: (510) 536-9929

American Chiropractic Association
1701 Clarendon Blvd.
Arlington, VA 22209
Tel: (800) 986-4636
memberinfo@amerchiro.org

American College of Rheumatology
1800 Century Place, Suite 250
Atlanta, GA 30345
Tel: (404) 633-3777
acr@rheumatology.org

American Council on Exercise (Pilates)
4851 Paramount Drive
San Diego, CA 92123
Tel: (800) 825-3636
Tel: (858) 279-8227

American Disability Association
Member Services
2201 Sixth Avenue South
Birmingham, Alabama 35233
Tel: (205) 328-9090

American Geriatrics Society
The Empire State Building
350 Fifth Avenue, Suite 801
New York, NY 10118
Tel: (212) 308-1414
Fax: 03 8699 0400
www.racgp.org.au

American Orthopaedic Association
6300 North River Road, Suite 505
Rosemont, IL 60018-4263
Tel: (847) 318-7330
info@aoaassn.org

American Osteopathic Association
142 East Ontario Street
Chicago, IL 60611
Tel: (800) 621-1773
Tel: (312) 202-8000

American Physical Therapy Association
1111 North Fairfax Street
Alexandria, VA 22314-1488
Tel: (800) 999-APTA
Tel: (703) 684-APTA

American Psychotherapy and Medical Hypnosis Association
1113 North Main Street
Weatherford, TX 76086
Tel: (817) 594-7003

American Society for the Alexander Technique
P.O. Box 60008
Florence, MA 01062
Tel: (800) 473-0620
Tel: (413) 584-2359
alexandertech@earthlink.net

Arthritis Foundation
CPR Department
1330 Peachtree Street
Atlanta, GA 30309
Tel: (800) 283-7800
Tel: (404) 872-7100

ErgoOutfitters.com
P.O. Box 64-3099
Vero Beach, FL 32963
Tel: (772) 492-5000

John Hopkins Arthritis Clinic
Bayview Medical Center
5501 Hopkins Bayview Circle
Baltimore, MD 21224
Tel: (410) 550-2400

**Mayo Clinic Health
Information Division**
200 First Street SW
Centerplace 5
Rochester, MN 55905

**National Center for
Complementary and
Alternative Medicine**
NCCAM Clearinghouse
P.O. Box 7923
Gaithersburg, MD 20898
Tel: (888) 644-6226

North American Spine Society
22 Calendar Court, 2nd floor
LaGrange, IL 60525
Tel: (877) SPINE-DR
info@spine.org

Relax the Back
(800) 222-5728

Safe Computing
1361 S. Winchester, Suite 107
San Jose, CA 95128
info@safecomputing.com

**Spondylitis Association of
America**
14827 Ventura Blvd. #222
Sherman Oaks, CA 91403
Tel: (800) 777-8189
Tel: (818) 981-1616
info@spondylitis.org
www.nrhp.co.uk

Canada

Acupuncture Canada
107 Leitch Drive
Grimbsy, ON L3M 2T9
Tel: (905) 563-8930
www.acupuncture.ca

The Arthritis Society
393 University Avenue,
Suite 1700
Toronto, ON M5G 1E6
Tel: (416) 979-7228
www.arthritis.ca

Canadian Back Institute
1243 Islington Avenue,
Suite 911
Toronto, ON M8X 1Y9
Tel: (416) 231-0078
www.cbi.ca

**Canadian Chiropractic
Association**
1396 Eglinton Avenue West
Toronto, ON M6C 2E4
Tel: (800) 668-2076
www.ccachiro.org

**Canadian College of
Osteopathy**
30 Duncan Street, Suite 701
Toronto, ON M5V 2C3
Tel: (416) 597-0367
www.osteopathy-canada.com

**Canadian Physiotherapy
Association**
2345 Yonge Street, Suite 410
Toronto, ON M4P 2E5
Tel: (800) 387-8679
www.physiotherapy.ca

**Canadian Rheumatology
Association**
43 Lundys Lane
Newmarket, ON L3Y 3R7
Tel: (905) 952-0698
www.cra-scr.ca

**Canadian Society of Teachers
of Alexander Technique**
465 Wilson Avenue
Toronto, ON M3H 1T9
Tel: (877) 598-8879
www.canstat.ca

Index

Acknowledgements

About the author

Dr. John Tanner is a private practitioner in orthopedic and sports medicine, with a special interest in back injuries and their treatment. He qualified in medicine and psychology in London and trained as a family doctor. He went on to study medical and osteopathic methods of manipulation, physical fitness training, rehabilitation of injured sportsmen, and pain management. He now runs a multidisciplinary clinic in the UK, specializing in musculoskeletal problems and also works at the BUPA Wellness Centre in London. A medical adviser to the Physical Medicine Research Foundation (Vancouver), Dr. Tanner is also on the Council of the British Institute of Musculoskeletal Medicine, and organizes the postgraduate teaching programme for doctors in this field.

Author's acknowledgements

Sincere thanks are due to my colleagues in the British Institute of Musculoskeletal Medicine and the Physical Medicine Research Foundation with whom I have held many interesting and productive discussions and meetings about back pain over the years. Thanks are also due to the many researchers around the world who each throw a little more light on the problem and help widen our understanding. Specifically I would like to thank Drs. Simon Blease and David Kay, radiologists, who have supplied some of the medical images, and Professor Ian Swain for his contribution on Moire Fringe topography. A warm thank you to my secretary Emma Dodd and staff for their help in compiling this book.

Publisher's acknowledgements

The publisher would like to thank: Dr. D. Lenrow from the Department of Rehabilitation at the University of Pennsylvania, USA, for advice; Dr. Marc White, Executive Director of the Physical Medicine Research Foundation of Vancouver for assistance; Hilary Bird for the index; Shannon Beatty for editorial assistance; Mark Cavanagh for design help; Cathy Meeus for the use of her garden.
Models Christopher James, Sarah Cookson, Amanda Grant, Elizabeth Howells, David Doma
Makeup Susie Kennett and Louise Heywood
Illustrators Philip Wilson, Simon Roulstone, John Woodcock and Nick Hall
Suppliers Keith Chittock, Huntleigh Akron, 1 Farthing Rd, Ipswich, Suffolk IP1 5AP
Michael Calver at The Back Shop, 14 New Cavendish Street, London W1M 7LJ
(Tel: 0207 935 9120) www.thebackshop.co.uk

Picture credits

Picture research Anna Bedewell
Picture library Claire Bowers, Romaine Werblow

The publisher would like to thank the following for kind permission to reproduce their photographs: (Abbreviations key: t=top, b=bottom, r=right, l=left) 54: Institute of Orthopaedics UCL (t), Science Photo Library/Zephyr (b). 58: Institute of Orthopaedics UCL (r). 78: Science Photo Library/Sovereign, ISM (l). 79: Medical Physics Dept. Salisbury, UK (b). 79: Dietrich Graf von Schweinitz.
All other images © Dorling Kindersley.
For further information see www.dkimages.com